STAGE 4 KIDNEY DISEASE DIET COOKBOOK FOR VEGANS

Easy-to-follow nutritious and delicious Renal-Friendly Recipes Low in Sodium, Phosphorus and Potassium. Includes 14 Days Meal Plan.

Olivia Endwell

Copyright Statement:

Disclaimer:

Individual results may vary, and the success of any dietary or lifestyle change depends on various factors, including but not limited to individual commitment and adherence. Before making significant changes to your diet or lifestyle, consult with a qualified healthcare professional

The views and opinions expressed in this book are those of the author and do not necessarily reflect the official policy or position of any other agency, organization, employer, or company.

TABLE OF CONTENTS

INTRODUCTION 1

Basics of vegan nutrition for kidney health 3

  Essential Nutrients for Kidney Function 3

  Vegan Protein Sources..4

  Managing Phosphorus and Potassium Intake 5

Tips and tricks for vegan cooking with kidney disease 6

  Flavoring without Adding Sodium 6

  Smart Substitutions for Restricted Ingredients..................7

  Cooking Techniques for Kidney-Friendly Meals 8

Vegan meal planning for stage 4 kidney disease.....................10

  Creating Balanced and Nutrient-Dense Meals 10

  Portion Control and Monitoring Fluid Intake....................12

Vegan grocery shopping and pantry essentials........................14

  Building a Kidney-Friendly Vegan Pantry 14

  Reading Food Labels for Phosphorus and Potassium 16

Salad Recipes 19

  1. Quinoa and Vegetable Salad...19

  2. Spinach and Chickpea Salad with Lemon Tahini Dressing......20

  3. Mango and Black Bean Quinoa Salad.............................22

4. Roasted Beet and Lentil Salad...24

5. Cauliflower and Broccoli Quinoa Bowl...............................25

6. Sweet Potato and Kale Salad with Avocado Dressing.............27

7. Cucumber and Chickpea Greek Salad.................................28

8. Rainbow Quinoa Salad with Citrus Dressing.......................30

9. Edamame and Asparagus Quinoa Salad..............................32

10. Avocado and Black Bean Salad with Lime-Cilantro Dressing

....33

Breakfast Recipes...36

1. Tofu Scramble with Spinach and Tomatoes 36

2. Oatmeal with Berries and Almond Butter 38

3. Avocado and Tomato Toast..39

4. Chia Seed Pudding with Mixed Fruit.................................41

5. Vegan Banana Walnut Pancakes.......................................42

6. Berry Smoothie Bowl...44

7. Vegan Tofu Pancakes with Blueberry Compote 45

8. Vegan Breakfast Burrito 47

9. Vegan Sweet Potato and Black Bean Hash..........................49

10. Vegan Spinach and Mushroom Frittata 50

11. Vegan Chia Seed Pancakes with Mixed Berry Compote........52

12. Vegan Tofu and Vegetable Breakfast Burrito 54

13. Vegan Quinoa Breakfast Bowl 56

14. Vegan Chickpea Flour Crepes with Berry Compote 57

15. Vegan Breakfast Quinoa Bowl with Almond Butter and Banana 59

16. Vegan Almond and Berry Breakfast Parfait 60

17. Vegan Chocolate Chia Seed Pudding 62

18. Vegan Blueberry and Almond Overnight Oats 63

19. Vegan Spinach and Mushroom Breakfast Wrap 64

20. Vegan Peanut Butter and Banana Toast 66

Lunch Recipes 68

1. Vegan Lentil and Vegetable Stew 68

2. Vegan Quinoa Salad with Chickpeas and Vegetables..............70

3. Vegan Chickpea and Spinach Curry 72

4. Vegan Mediterranean Quinoa Bowl 73

5. Vegan Sweet Potato and Black Bean Burrito Bowl..................75

6. Vegan Roasted Vegetable and Quinoa Salad 77

7. Vegan Black Bean and Corn Quesadillas 79

8. Vegan Eggplant and Tomato Pasta 81

9. Vegan Butternut Squash and Kale Salad 82

10. Vegan Cauliflower and Chickpea Curry...................................84

11. Vegan Spinach and Mushroom Stuffed Bell Peppers 85

12. Vegan Sweet and Spicy Tofu Stir-Fry 87

13. Vegan Zucchini Noodles with Pesto 89

14. Vegan Lentil and Vegetable Stir-Fry 90

15. Vegan Stuffed Bell Peppers with Quinoa and Black Beans ... 92

16. Vegan Chickpea and Vegetable Stir-Fry 94

17. Vegan Mediterranean Chickpea Salad 95

18. Vegan Avocado and Chickpea Wrap 97

19. Vegan Roasted Red Pepper and Hummus Sandwich 99

20. Vegan Broccoli and Almond Stir-Fry 100

Dinner Recipes 103

1. Vegan Chickpea and Vegetable Curry 103

2. Vegan Lentil and Mushroom Stuffed Peppers 105

3. Vegan Quinoa and Vegetable Stir-Fry 107

4. Vegan Spaghetti with Lentil Bolognese 108

5. Vegan Sweet Potato and Black Bean Chili 110

6. Vegan Cauliflower and Chickpea Curry 112

7. Vegan Stuffed Portobello Mushrooms 113

8. Vegan Mediterranean Couscous Salad 115

9. Vegan Black Bean and Quinoa Stuffed Bell Peppers 117

10. Vegan Eggplant and Chickpea Tagine 118

11. Vegan Spinach and Artichoke Stuffed Mushrooms 120

12. Vegan Teriyaki Tofu and Vegetable Skewers 122

13. Vegan Butternut Squash and Lentil Stew 124

14. Vegan Mediterranean Stuffed Acorn Squash......................125

15. Vegan Mushroom and Spinach Risotto 127

16. Vegan Chickpea and Spinach Quesadillas..........................129

17. Vegan Teriyaki Vegetable and Tofu Stir-Fry 131

18. Vegan Quinoa and Black Bean Bowl 133

19. Vegan Lentil and Vegetable Curry 134

20. Vegan Spicy Black Bean and Sweet Potato Enchiladas 136

Snack Recipes 139

1. Vegan Avocado and Black Bean Dip..................................139

2. Vegan Roasted Chickpeas...140

3. Vegan Cucumber and Hummus Bites..................................142

4. Vegan Stuffed Bell Pepper Poppers...................................143

5. Vegan Edamame and Sea Salt 144

6. Vegan Sweet Potato Chips...145

7. Vegan Berry and Almond Parfait.......................................146

8. Vegan Kale Chips 148

9. Vegan Banana and Walnut Oat Bars..................................149

10. Vegan Mango Salsa with Jicama Chips............................150

14-Day Meal Plan 152

Lifestyle strategies for managing kidney disease 157

Incorporating Physical Activity for Kidney Health....................157

Stress Management and Kidney Health 158

Regular Monitoring and Consultation with Healthcare

Professionals...159

Conclusion 162

INTRODUCTION

Welcome to the journey of nourishing your body and embracing a plant-based lifestyle tailored specifically for managing Stage 4 kidney disease. In this guide, we'll delve into the intricacies of understanding your condition and highlight the crucial role a vegan diet can play in promoting kidney health.

Firstly, let's unravel the mysteries surrounding Stage 4 Kidney Disease. It's a stage where kidney function is significantly impaired, demanding a nuanced approach to dietary choices. As your kidneys work tirelessly to filter out waste and excess fluids, understanding the intricacies of this condition becomes paramount. We'll explore the challenges it presents and equip you with insights to make informed decisions about your diet and overall well-being.

Now, let's address the powerful ally in your journey: a vegan diet. Many might wonder, why vegan? The answer lies in the unique advantages it brings to the table. A well-planned vegan diet can be a cornerstone in managing kidney disease, offering a plethora of plant-based nutrients that support renal function. We'll explore the benefits of choosing plant-powered nourishment, providing you with a roadmap to delicious and kidney-friendly meals.

So, whether you're a seasoned vegan or someone embarking on a plant-based lifestyle for the first time, join us in discovering how mindful nutrition can be a transformative force in navigating Stage 4

Kidney Disease. Let's embark on this journey together, where each recipe, each tip, and each piece of knowledge becomes a stepping stone toward a healthier and more vibrant life.

BASICS OF VEGAN NUTRITION FOR KIDNEY HEALTH

Essential Nutrients for Kidney Function

Navigating Stage 4 Kidney Disease requires a thoughtful consideration of essential nutrients that contribute to overall kidney health. These nutrients act as building blocks for optimal function and play a crucial role in supporting your body's filtration system.

Protein is a fundamental nutrient, but it's imperative to choose the right sources in a vegan diet. Plant-based proteins such as beans, lentils, and tofu can be excellent choices. These sources not only provide essential amino acids but also come with the added benefit of being lower in phosphorus, a vital consideration for kidney health.

Ensuring an adequate intake of omega-3 fatty acids is another key element. While fatty fish is a typical source, vegan alternatives like chia seeds, flaxseeds, and walnuts can offer these heart-healthy fats. Omega-3s contribute to reducing inflammation and promoting cardiovascular health, factors crucial for those with compromised kidney function.

Vitamins and minerals, such as B-complex vitamins, vitamin C, and iron, are essential for maintaining energy levels and supporting overall health. Incorporating a variety of fruits, vegetables, and whole grains into your diet can help meet these nutritional needs. However, it's crucial to balance these choices to manage potential excesses in certain minerals, a common concern for those with kidney issues.

Vegan Protein Sources

Protein, often considered the cornerstone of a healthy diet, takes center stage in the context of kidney health. For those adhering to a vegan lifestyle, sourcing protein becomes a mindful task, requiring a diverse approach to meet nutritional requirements without overloading on phosphorus and potassium.

Legumes, including beans, lentils, and chickpeas, stand out as versatile and kidney-friendly protein sources. Rich in fiber and low in phosphorus and potassium, they contribute essential amino acids without placing undue stress on the kidneys. Tofu and tempeh, derived from soybeans, offer additional protein options with the added benefit of being adaptable to various culinary styles.

Nuts and seeds, such as almonds, pumpkin seeds, and hemp seeds, not only provide protein but also deliver heart-healthy fats and essential minerals. While they add a satisfying crunch to meals, it's essential to be mindful of portion sizes to manage phosphorus intake effectively.

Whole grains, including quinoa, brown rice, and oats, contribute both protein and fiber, making them valuable components of a kidney-friendly vegan diet. These grains offer a wholesome base for various dishes, from breakfast bowls to hearty dinners, providing a nutritional boost without compromising kidney function.

Managing Phosphorus and Potassium Intake

Phosphorus and potassium management becomes a pivotal aspect of dietary planning for those with Stage 4 Kidney Disease. These minerals, while essential, require careful consideration to prevent imbalances that may exacerbate kidney issues.

Phosphorus, abundant in many foods, poses a challenge for individuals with compromised kidney function. Plant-based sources of phosphorus, such as nuts, seeds, and whole grains, are healthier choices compared to processed foods. However, moderation is key, and understanding how to balance these foods within your daily intake is crucial. Soaking and cooking methods can be employed to reduce phosphorus levels in certain foods, enhancing their kidney-friendly profile.

Potassium, vital for nerve and muscle function, requires a delicate balance. Fruits and vegetables are rich in potassium, and including a variety of these in your diet is essential. However, knowledge of individual tolerances and incorporating cooking techniques like boiling or leaching can help manage potassium levels effectively. Identifying low-potassium alternatives ensures a well-rounded diet without compromising kidney health.

TIPS AND TRICKS FOR VEGAN COOKING WITH KIDNEY DISEASE

Embarking on a vegan journey while managing Stage 4 Kidney Disease opens a world of culinary possibilities. To navigate this path successfully, it's essential to master the art of vegan cooking tailored to kidney health. In this chapter, we'll explore invaluable tips and tricks that will not only tantalize your taste buds but also support your overall well-being.

Flavoring without Adding Sodium

One of the most common challenges for individuals with kidney disease is managing sodium intake. While sodium is a ubiquitous flavor enhancer, there are numerous ways to infuse depth into your vegan dishes without relying on salt.

Herbs and spices become your culinary allies in this quest. Fresh herbs like basil, cilantro, and parsley add vibrancy and freshness to your meals without contributing to sodium concerns. Dried spices such as cumin, paprika, and turmeric not only bring robust flavors but also offer additional health benefits. Experimenting with different herb and spice combinations allows you to create a diverse array of dishes while keeping sodium levels in check.

Citrus fruits, such as lemons and limes, provide a zesty burst of flavor without the need for salt. Incorporating citrus-based dressings or marinades not only elevates the taste of your dishes but also adds a refreshing twist. Additionally, vinegars, like balsamic or apple cider vinegar, can be used judiciously to enhance the acidity and complexity of your meals.

Umami-rich ingredients, such as nutritional yeast, miso paste, and tamari (a low-sodium soy sauce alternative), introduce savory notes to your recipes. These flavor enhancers contribute depth without compromising kidney health. Nutritional yeast, in particular, adds a cheesy flavor, making it an excellent substitute for dairy in vegan recipes.

Smart Substitutions for Restricted Ingredients

Adapting to a vegan diet for kidney health often involves smart substitutions to replace ingredients that may pose challenges. Whether it's finding alternatives to high-potassium vegetables or replacing phosphorus-rich components, thoughtful choices can make a significant difference.

Potatoes, a staple in many diets, can be swapped for lower-potassium alternatives like sweet potatoes or cauliflower. These alternatives not only provide a similar texture but also offer unique flavors and nutritional benefits. Likewise, exploring a variety of grains beyond traditional wheat can open up new possibilities. Buckwheat, quinoa, and millet are nutrient-rich alternatives that bring diversity to your plate.

Dairy replacements are a crucial aspect of vegan cooking, and for those with kidney disease, choosing wisely is essential. Plant-based milk options such as almond, rice, or oat milk can be suitable alternatives, but it's crucial to opt for unsweetened varieties to avoid unnecessary sugars. Experimenting with different plant-based yogurts and cheeses allows you to discover alternatives that align with your dietary restrictions while adding creaminess and flavor to your dishes.

Protein sources also demand careful consideration. While beans and lentils are excellent choices, managing phosphorus levels might require exploring protein alternatives. Seitan, a high-protein meat substitute made from gluten, can be a valuable addition to your repertoire. Tofu and tempeh, derived from soybeans, offer versatile and kidney-friendly protein options.

Cooking Techniques for Kidney-Friendly Meals

Beyond ingredient selection, mastering kidney-friendly cooking techniques is a key element of crafting delicious vegan meals. How you prepare your food can impact its nutrient content and overall suitability for kidney health.

Boiling and soaking are effective methods for reducing phosphorus content in certain foods. For instance, soaking beans and legumes before cooking can help leach out some of the phosphorus, making them more kidney-friendly. Additionally, boiling vegetables can be a practical way to manage potassium levels, as some of the potassium leaches into the cooking water.

Grilling and roasting add depth and flavor to your dishes without compromising kidney health. These techniques enhance the natural sugars in vegetables, providing a caramelized exterior and a tender interior. Roasting, in particular, intensifies flavors and textures, making it an excellent method for preparing a variety of plant-based dishes.

Stir-frying is a quick and efficient way to cook vegetables while preserving their nutritional content. Using heart-healthy oils, such as olive oil, contributes to the overall well-being of your kidneys. Opting for a variety of colorful vegetables not only makes your stir-fry visually appealing but also ensures a diverse range of nutrients.

Steaming is a gentle cooking method that retains the maximum amount of nutrients in your food. This technique is especially useful for vegetables, preserving their crispness and vibrant colors. Steaming also requires minimal added fats, making it a heart-healthy option for those with kidney concerns.

VEGAN MEAL PLANNING FOR STAGE 4 KIDNEY DISEASE

Embarking on a vegan lifestyle while managing Stage 4 Kidney Disease requires a thoughtful and strategic approach to meal planning. In this chapter, we'll delve into two critical aspects: creating balanced and nutrient-dense meals and mastering portion control while vigilantly monitoring fluid intake.

Creating Balanced and Nutrient-Dense Meals

Balancing a vegan diet for optimal kidney health involves a meticulous selection of foods to ensure a comprehensive range of nutrients while considering the limitations imposed by Stage 4 Kidney Disease. Here, we explore the key principles of crafting balanced and nutrient-dense vegan meals that nourish your body while supporting renal function.

Diversity of Plant-Based Foods: The cornerstone of a balanced vegan diet for kidney health lies in the diversity of plant-based foods. By incorporating a wide range of fruits, vegetables, whole grains, legumes, and nuts, you ensure a spectrum of essential vitamins, minerals, and antioxidants. This diversity not only provides a rich tapestry of flavors but also contributes to the overall well-being of your kidneys.

Mindful Protein Selection: Protein is an essential component of any diet, and for those with Stage 4 Kidney Disease, opting for high-quality vegan protein sources becomes crucial. Beans, lentils, tofu, tempeh, and edamame are excellent choices that offer a complete amino acid profile. Balancing these protein sources with a variety of grains and vegetables ensures that you receive the full spectrum of essential amino acids necessary for optimal health.

Strategic Nutrient Considerations: Navigating the intricacies of nutrient intake becomes paramount. While some nutrients need to be moderated, others must be carefully ensured. Phosphorus and potassium, in particular, require attention. By choosing low-phosphorus plant-based foods and balancing high-potassium items, you can create meals that align with kidney health recommendations. Careful planning ensures that nutrient restrictions do not compromise the overall nutritional value of your meals.

Incorporating Healthy Fats: Healthy fats play a vital role in a well-rounded diet, contributing to overall health and satiety. Avocados, nuts, seeds, and olive oil are excellent sources of heart-healthy fats that can be incorporated into your vegan meals. These fats not only enhance the flavor and texture of your dishes but also support nutrient absorption, contributing to the overall efficacy of your kidney-friendly diet.

Monitoring Sodium Intake: Sodium management is a critical consideration for individuals with kidney disease. While a vegan diet inherently tends to be lower in sodium than an omnivorous one, it's essential to be mindful of additional sources. Choosing fresh, whole foods over processed options and flavoring your meals with herbs and spices rather than salt are effective strategies to control sodium intake. By prioritizing these choices, you can create flavorful meals without compromising kidney health.

Portion Control and Monitoring Fluid Intake

Beyond the selection of foods, mastering portion control and monitoring fluid intake are vital components of effective vegan meal planning for Stage 4 Kidney Disease. These aspects ensure that you strike the right balance, providing nourishment without overburdening your kidneys.

Portion Control Strategies: Portion control is a key element in managing nutrient intake, especially for those with kidney disease. While plant-based foods are generally nutrient-dense, it's crucial to be mindful of portion sizes to avoid overconsumption. Measuring and weighing ingredients, using smaller plates, and paying attention to hunger and fullness cues can all contribute to effective portion control.

Balancing Macronutrients: Achieving a balance of macronutrients—proteins, carbohydrates, and fats—is essential for overall health and kidney function. Carefully considering the distribution of these macronutrients in your meals helps prevent excessive intake of certain components. For example, while carbohydrates are an important energy source, balancing them with proteins and healthy fats helps stabilize blood sugar levels and supports sustained energy.

Fluid Intake Management: Monitoring fluid intake is a critical aspect of kidney disease management. While hydration is essential, individuals with compromised kidney function must be vigilant about not overloading the system. Consulting with a healthcare professional to determine a suitable daily fluid limit is a crucial first step. Additionally, considering not just the liquids you drink but also the water content in fruits and vegetables is essential for accurate fluid management.

Strategic Meal Timing: Meal timing can impact how your body processes nutrients and manages fluid levels. Spreading your meals throughout the day and avoiding large, heavy meals close to bedtime can help regulate nutrient absorption and reduce the risk of fluid overload. Strategic meal timing also contributes to stable blood sugar levels and supports overall kidney health.

Recordkeeping and Monitoring: Maintaining a food diary can be a valuable tool for tracking your dietary choices, portion sizes, and fluid intake. Regular monitoring allows you to identify patterns, make informed adjustments, and collaborate effectively with healthcare professionals to optimize your vegan meal plan for Stage 4 Kidney Disease.

VEGAN GROCERY SHOPPING AND PANTRY ESSENTIALS

Embarking on a vegan lifestyle while managing Stage 4 Kidney Disease involves not only thoughtful meal planning but also strategic grocery shopping and maintaining a well-stocked pantry. In this chapter, we will explore the essentials of building a kidney-friendly vegan pantry and mastering the art of reading food labels, with a specific focus on phosphorus and potassium content.

Building a Kidney-Friendly Vegan Pantry

Creating a kidney-friendly vegan pantry requires a blend of foresight, knowledge, and intentional selection. By stocking up on the right ingredients, you set the foundation for preparing wholesome and nourishing meals that align with the dietary restrictions imposed by Stage 4 Kidney Disease.

Low-Phosphorus Staples: Phosphorus management is a key consideration for those with kidney disease. Building a kidney-friendly vegan pantry involves selecting staples that are naturally low in phosphorus. Whole grains like brown rice and quinoa, which are lower in phosphorus compared to their refined counterparts, serve as excellent pantry staples. Additionally, choosing pasta made from alternative flours such as lentil or chickpea flour can provide variety while remaining phosphorus-conscious.

Phosphorus-Aware Proteins: Proteins are essential for a balanced vegan diet, but for those managing kidney disease, selecting phosphorus-aware protein sources is crucial. Stock your pantry with dried beans and lentils, opting for the low-phosphorus varieties. Canned beans, after thorough rinsing, can also be a convenient and kidney-friendly protein source. Tofu and tempeh, derived from soybeans, are versatile and protein-rich additions that align well with kidney health goals.

Nuts and Seeds in Moderation: Nuts and seeds add texture, flavor, and healthy fats to vegan meals, but they can also be significant sources of phosphorus. Almonds, chia seeds, and flaxseeds are popular choices with nutritional benefits, but moderation is key. By incorporating these items into your pantry in controlled quantities, you can enjoy their benefits without compromising phosphorus levels.

Low-Potassium Alternatives: Potassium management is another essential aspect of a kidney-friendly vegan pantry. Selecting low-potassium alternatives ensures that you can enjoy a variety of flavors without exceeding recommended potassium levels. Opt for vegetables like bell peppers, cauliflower, and zucchini, which are lower in potassium compared to high-potassium counterparts. Choosing fruits such as apples, berries, and peaches also contributes to a kidney-conscious pantry.

Dried Herbs and Spices: Flavoring your meals without relying on sodium becomes an art in kidney-friendly cooking. Dried herbs and spices are invaluable pantry staples that not only enhance the taste of your dishes but also provide numerous health benefits. Stock up on options like thyme, oregano, cumin, and turmeric to add depth to your meals without compromising kidney health.

Whole-Grain Flours: If baking is part of your culinary repertoire, incorporating whole-grain flours like oat flour, brown rice flour, or chickpea flour can provide a nutrient-dense alternative to traditional refined flours. These options not only contribute to a healthier pantry but also support kidney-conscious meal preparation.

Reading Food Labels for Phosphorus and Potassium

Navigating the grocery store aisles becomes a skill when managing Stage 4 Kidney Disease. Understanding how to read food labels, specifically focusing on phosphorus and potassium content, empowers individuals to make informed choices that align with their dietary restrictions.

Understanding Serving Sizes: One of the first steps in deciphering food labels is understanding serving sizes. The nutrient content listed on the label is often based on a specific serving size, and this information is crucial for accurate assessment. Paying attention to serving sizes ensures that you can gauge the phosphorus and potassium intake more precisely, preventing unintentional overconsumption.

Checking for Additives: Processed and packaged foods may contain additives that can contribute to increased phosphorus and potassium levels. Ingredients like phosphates and potassium-based additives may be listed under various names. Being vigilant about checking for these additives on food labels allows you to make choices that align with kidney-friendly guidelines.

Differentiating Between Phosphorus Forms: Phosphorus exists in various forms, and not all forms are equally absorbed by the body. Understanding the distinction between organic and inorganic phosphorus can be crucial. While organic phosphorus is naturally occurring and less readily absorbed, inorganic phosphorus, often found in additives, is more easily absorbed. By discerning between these forms, you can make choices that mitigate phosphorus-related concerns.

Identifying Hidden Potassium: Potassium content can be stealthily concealed in certain food items. Reading food labels attentively helps in identifying sources of hidden potassium. For instance, certain low-sodium products may use potassium-based substitutes, and familiarizing yourself with these nuances aids in making choices that align with your kidney health goals.

Comparing Brands and Products: Not all brands or product variations are created equal when it comes to phosphorus and potassium content. Comparing different brands and product options enables you to make selections that are more tailored to your dietary restrictions. Opting for lower phosphorus and potassium alternatives within a category provides flexibility without compromising on taste.

Utilizing Apps and Resources: In the digital age, several apps and online resources are specifically designed to assist individuals with kidney disease in managing their dietary choices. These tools allow you to scan barcodes, access nutritional information, and make on-the-spot decisions while grocery shopping. Incorporating these resources into your shopping routine adds an extra layer of support to your kidney-conscious lifestyle.

SALAD RECIPES

1. Quinoa and Vegetable Salad

Prep Time: 15 minutes

Cooking Time: 15 minutes

Serving Size: 2

Ingredients:

- 1 cup cooked quinoa
- 1 cup cherry tomatoes, halved
- 1 cucumber, diced
- 1/2 red onion, finely chopped
- 1/4 cup fresh parsley, chopped
- 2 tablespoons olive oil
- 1 tablespoon balsamic vinegar
- Salt and pepper to taste

Instructions:

1. In a large bowl, combine the cooked quinoa, cherry tomatoes, cucumber, red onion, and fresh parsley.

2. In a small bowl, whisk together the olive oil and balsamic vinegar. Season with salt and pepper.

3. Pour the dressing over the quinoa mixture and toss well to coat.

4. Allow the salad to marinate for at least 10 minutes before serving.

5. Serve chilled and enjoy a kidney-friendly, nutrient-packed meal!

Nutritional Information (per serving):

- Calories: 320

- Protein: 8g

- Carbohydrates: 45g

- Fiber: 7g

- Potassium: 350mg

- Phosphorus: 150mg

2. Spinach and Chickpea Salad with Lemon Tahini Dressing

Prep Time: 20 minutes

Cooking Time: 0 minutes

Serving Size: 2

Ingredients:

- 4 cups fresh spinach leaves

- 1 can (15 oz) chickpeas, drained and rinsed

- 1 cup cherry tomatoes, halved

- 1/4 cup red bell pepper, diced

- 2 tablespoons tahini

- 2 tablespoons lemon juice

- 1 tablespoon water

- 1 clove garlic, minced

- Salt and pepper to taste

Instructions:

1. In a large salad bowl, combine the fresh spinach, chickpeas, cherry tomatoes, and red bell pepper.

2. In a separate bowl, whisk together tahini, lemon juice, water, minced garlic, salt, and pepper to create the dressing.

3. Pour the dressing over the salad and toss until well coated.

4. Allow the flavors to meld for 10 minutes before serving.

5. This refreshing salad is rich in plant-based protein and kidney-friendly nutrients.

Nutritional Information (per serving):

- Calories: 320

- Protein: 12g

- Carbohydrates: 40g

- Fiber: 10g

- Potassium: 400mg

- Phosphorus: 180mg

3. Mango and Black Bean Quinoa Salad

Prep Time: 20 minutes

Cooking Time: 15 minutes

Serving Size: 2

Ingredients:

- 1 cup cooked quinoa

- 1 ripe mango, diced

- 1 can (15 oz) black beans, drained and rinsed

- 1/2 red onion, finely chopped

- 1/4 cup fresh cilantro, chopped

- 2 tablespoons lime juice

- 1 tablespoon olive oil

- Salt and cayenne pepper to taste

Instructions:

1. In a large mixing bowl, combine the cooked quinoa, diced mango, black beans, red onion, and fresh cilantro.

2. In a small bowl, whisk together lime juice, olive oil, salt, and cayenne pepper to create the dressing.

3. Pour the dressing over the salad and toss gently until well combined.

4. Allow the salad to chill for 15 minutes before serving.

5. Enjoy the vibrant flavors of this kidney-friendly vegan salad!

Nutritional Information (per serving):

- Calories: 340

- Protein: 9g

- Carbohydrates: 55g

- Fiber: 11g

- Potassium: 380mg

- Phosphorus: 200mg

4. Roasted Beet and Lentil Salad

Prep Time: 25 minutes

Cooking Time: 30 minutes

Serving Size: 2

Ingredients:

- 2 medium-sized beets, roasted and diced

- 1 cup cooked green lentils

- 1 cup arugula

- 1/4 cup red onion, thinly sliced

- 2 tablespoons balsamic vinegar

- 1 tablespoon olive oil

- 1 teaspoon Dijon mustard

- Salt and pepper to taste

Instructions:

1. Preheat the oven to 400°F (200°C). Wrap beets in foil and roast until tender (about 30 minutes). Allow to cool, peel, and dice.

2. In a salad bowl, combine roasted beets, cooked lentils, arugula, and sliced red onion.

3. In a small bowl, whisk together balsamic vinegar, olive oil, Dijon mustard, salt, and pepper to create the dressing.

4. Drizzle the dressing over the salad and toss gently to coat.

5. Let the flavors meld for 15 minutes before serving this nutrient-packed vegan dish.

Nutritional Information (per serving):

- Calories: 310

- Protein: 14g

- Carbohydrates: 45g

- Fiber: 12g

- Potassium: 520mg

- Phosphorus: 240mg

5. Cauliflower and Broccoli Quinoa Bowl

Prep Time: 20 minutes

Cooking Time: 20 minutes

Serving Size: 2

Ingredients:

- 1 cup cooked quinoa

- 1 cup cauliflower florets

- 1 cup broccoli florets

- 1/4 cup sun-dried tomatoes, chopped

- 2 tablespoons olive oil

- 1 tablespoon lemon juice

- 1 teaspoon dried thyme

- Salt and pepper to taste

Instructions:

1. In a large bowl, mix the cooked quinoa, cauliflower florets, broccoli florets, and sun-dried tomatoes.

2. In a small bowl, whisk together olive oil, lemon juice, dried thyme, salt, and pepper to create the dressing.

3. Drizzle the dressing over the quinoa mixture and toss gently until well coated.

4. Allow the salad to marinate for 10 minutes before serving.

5. This kidney-friendly vegan bowl is a tasty combination of textures and flavors.

Nutritional Information (per serving):

- Calories: 330

- Protein: 10g

- Carbohydrates: 50g

- Fiber: 8g

- Potassium: 400mg

- Phosphorus: 180mg

6. Sweet Potato and Kale Salad with Avocado Dressing

Prep Time: 25 minutes

Cooking Time: 30 minutes

Serving Size: 2

Ingredients:

- 1 large sweet potato, peeled and diced

- 2 cups kale, chopped

- 1/4 cup red onion, finely chopped

- 1/2 avocado

- 2 tablespoons lime juice

- 1 tablespoon olive oil

- 1 teaspoon maple syrup

- Salt and pepper to taste

Instructions:

1. Preheat the oven to 400°F (200°C). Roast the sweet potato cubes until tender (about 30 minutes).

2. In a large bowl, combine roasted sweet potatoes, chopped kale, and red onion.

3. In a blender, blend together avocado, lime juice, olive oil, maple syrup, salt, and pepper to create the dressing.

4. Pour the avocado dressing over the salad and toss gently until well combined.

5. Let the salad sit for 10 minutes before serving this nutrient-rich and kidney-friendly dish.

Nutritional Information (per serving):

- Calories: 340

- Protein: 8g

- Carbohydrates: 50g

- Fiber: 10g

- Potassium: 420mg

- Phosphorus: 200mg

7. Cucumber and Chickpea Greek Salad

Prep Time: 15 minutes

Cooking Time: 0 minutes

Serving Size: 2

Ingredients:

- 1 cucumber, diced

- 1 can (15 oz) chickpeas, drained and rinsed

- 1 cup cherry tomatoes, halved

- 1/4 cup red onion, finely chopped

- 1/2 cup Kalamata olives, sliced

- 1/4 cup fresh parsley, chopped

- 2 tablespoons olive oil

- 2 tablespoons red wine vinegar

- 1 teaspoon dried oregano

- Salt and pepper to taste

Instructions:

1. In a large salad bowl, combine diced cucumber, chickpeas, cherry tomatoes, red onion, sliced olives, and fresh parsley.

2. In a small bowl, whisk together olive oil, red wine vinegar, dried oregano, salt, and pepper to create the dressing.

3. Pour the dressing over the salad and toss gently until well coated.

4. Allow the flavors to meld for 10 minutes before serving this refreshing and kidney-friendly Greek salad.

Nutritional Information (per serving):

- Calories: 320

- Protein: 9g

- Carbohydrates: 45g

- Fiber: 12g

- Potassium: 380mg

- Phosphorus: 220mg

8. Rainbow Quinoa Salad with Citrus Dressing

Prep Time: 20 minutes

Cooking Time: 15 minutes

Serving Size: 2

Ingredients:

- 1 cup cooked rainbow quinoa

- 1 cup shredded purple cabbage

- 1 carrot, julienned

- 1/2 bell pepper (any color), diced

- 1/4 cup raisins

- 2 tablespoons pumpkin seeds

- 2 tablespoons orange juice

- 1 tablespoon olive oil

- 1 teaspoon Dijon mustard

- Salt and pepper to taste

Instructions:

1. In a large bowl, combine cooked quinoa, shredded purple cabbage, julienned carrot, diced bell pepper, raisins, and pumpkin seeds.

2. In a small bowl, whisk together orange juice, olive oil, Dijon mustard, salt, and pepper to create the dressing.

3. Drizzle the dressing over the salad and toss gently until well coated.

4. Allow the salad to marinate for 15 minutes before serving this vibrant and nutrient-packed dish.

Nutritional Information (per serving):

- Calories: 330

- Protein: 9g

- Carbohydrates: 50g

- Fiber: 8g

- Potassium: 400mg

- Phosphorus: 180mg

9. Edamame and Asparagus Quinoa Salad

Prep Time: 25 minutes

Cooking Time: 15 minutes

Serving Size: 2

Ingredients:

- 1 cup cooked quinoa

- 1 cup edamame, shelled

- 1 cup asparagus, chopped

- 1/4 cup red bell pepper, diced

- 2 tablespoons sesame oil

- 1 tablespoon soy sauce (low-sodium)

- 1 tablespoon rice vinegar

- 1 teaspoon maple syrup

- Sesame seeds for garnish

Instructions:

1. In a large bowl, combine cooked quinoa, shelled edamame, chopped asparagus, and diced red bell pepper.

2. In a small bowl, whisk together sesame oil, low-sodium soy sauce, rice vinegar, and maple syrup to create the dressing.

3. Pour the dressing over the salad and toss gently until well coated.

4. Garnish with sesame seeds and let the salad sit for 10 minutes before serving this protein-packed and kidney-friendly dish.

Nutritional Information (per serving):

- Calories: 340

- Protein: 13g

- Carbohydrates: 45g

- Fiber: 9g

- Potassium: 420mg

- Phosphorus: 200mg

10. Avocado and Black Bean Salad with Lime-Cilantro Dressing

Prep Time: 20 minutes
Cooking Time: 0 minutes
Serving Size: 2

Ingredients:

- 1 can (15 oz) black beans, drained and rinsed

- 1 avocado, diced

- 1 cup corn kernels (fresh or frozen)

- 1/4 cup red onion, finely chopped

- 2 tablespoons fresh cilantro, chopped

- 2 tablespoons lime juice

- 1 tablespoon olive oil

- 1 teaspoon cumin

- Salt and pepper to taste

Instructions:

1. In a large salad bowl, combine black beans, diced avocado, corn kernels, chopped red onion, and fresh cilantro.

2. In a small bowl, whisk together lime juice, olive oil, cumin, salt, and pepper to create the dressing.

3. Pour the dressing over the salad and toss gently until well coated.

4. Allow the salad to chill for 15 minutes before serving this flavorful and kidney-friendly dish.

Nutritional Information (per serving):

- Calories: 340

- Protein: 10g

- Carbohydrates: 50g

- Fiber: 13g

- Potassium: 410mg

- Phosphorus: 180mg

BREAKFAST RECIPES

1. Tofu Scramble with Spinach and Tomatoes

Prep Time: 10 minutes

Cooking Time: 15 minutes

Serving Size: 2

Ingredients:

- 1 block firm tofu, crumbled

- 2 cups fresh spinach, chopped

- 1 cup cherry tomatoes, halved

- 1/4 cup red onion, diced

- 1 tablespoon nutritional yeast

- 1 tablespoon olive oil

- 1 teaspoon turmeric powder

- Salt and pepper to taste

Instructions:

1. In a skillet, heat olive oil over medium heat. Add diced red onion and sauté until translucent.

2. Add crumbled tofu to the skillet, along with turmeric powder, salt, and pepper. Cook for 5-7 minutes until tofu is lightly browned.

3. Stir in chopped spinach and cherry tomatoes. Cook for an additional 3-5 minutes until spinach is wilted and tomatoes are softened.

4. Sprinkle nutritional yeast over the tofu scramble and toss to combine.

5. Serve hot, providing a protein-rich and kidney-friendly start to your day.

Nutritional Information (per serving):

- Calories: 220

- Protein: 18g

- Carbohydrates: 10g

- Fiber: 4g

- Potassium: 400mg

- Phosphorus: 180mg

2. Oatmeal with Berries and Almond Butter

Prep Time: 5 minutes

Cooking Time: 10 minutes

Serving Size: 1

Ingredients:

- 1/2 cup old-fashioned oats

- 1 cup unsweetened almond milk

- 1/2 cup mixed berries (blueberries, strawberries, raspberries)

- 1 tablespoon almond butter

- 1 tablespoon chia seeds

- 1 teaspoon maple syrup (optional)

- 1/2 teaspoon vanilla extract

Instructions:

1. In a saucepan, combine oats and almond milk. Cook over medium heat, stirring frequently, until the oats are creamy.

2. Stir in vanilla extract and chia seeds, continuing to cook for an additional 2-3 minutes.

3. Transfer the oatmeal to a bowl and top with mixed berries and a dollop of almond butter.

4. Drizzle with maple syrup if desired. Enjoy this nutrient-packed and kidney-friendly breakfast.

Nutritional Information (per serving):

- Calories: 350

- Protein: 12g

- Carbohydrates: 45g

- Fiber: 10g

- Potassium: 280mg

- Phosphorus: 180mg

3. Avocado and Tomato Toast

Prep Time: 5 minutes

Cooking Time: 5 minutes

Serving Size: 1

Ingredients:

- 1 slice whole-grain bread

- 1/2 avocado, mashed

- 1 medium tomato, sliced

- 1 teaspoon lemon juice

- Sprinkle of black pepper

- Fresh basil leaves for garnish

Instructions:

1. Toast the whole-grain bread to your desired level of crispiness.

2. Spread mashed avocado evenly over the toasted bread.

3. Arrange sliced tomatoes on top of the avocado.

4. Drizzle lemon juice over the tomatoes and sprinkle with black pepper.

5. Garnish with fresh basil leaves for added flavor and serve. This simple yet satisfying breakfast is kidney-friendly and full of healthy fats.

Nutritional Information (per serving):

- Calories: 250

- Protein: 6g

- Carbohydrates: 30g

- Fiber: 9g

- Potassium: 450mg

- Phosphorus: 150mg

4. Chia Seed Pudding with Mixed Fruit

Prep Time: 5 minutes (plus overnight refrigeration)

Cooking Time: 0 minutes

Serving Size: 1

Ingredients:

- 2 tablespoons chia seeds

- 1/2 cup unsweetened almond milk

- 1/2 teaspoon vanilla extract

- 1 tablespoon maple syrup

- 1/2 cup mixed fruit (berries, kiwi, pineapple)

Instructions:

1. In a bowl, mix chia seeds, almond milk, vanilla extract, and maple syrup. Stir well and refrigerate overnight.

2. In the morning, give the chia pudding a good stir.

3. Layer the chia pudding with mixed fruit in a serving glass.

4. Garnish with additional fruit on top and enjoy this refreshing and kidney-friendly breakfast.

Nutritional Information (per serving):

- Calories: 230

- Protein: 5g

- Carbohydrates: 35g

- Fiber: 10g

- Potassium: 280mg

- Phosphorus: 120mg

5. Vegan Banana Walnut Pancakes

Prep Time: 10 minutes

Cooking Time: 15 minutes

Serving Size: 2

Ingredients:

- 1 cup whole wheat flour

- 1 tablespoon flaxseed meal

- 1 teaspoon baking powder

- 1/2 teaspoon cinnamon

- 1 ripe banana, mashed

- 1 cup almond milk

- 1/4 cup chopped walnuts

- 1 teaspoon vanilla extract

- 1 tablespoon maple syrup (optional)

Instructions:

1. In a bowl, whisk together whole wheat flour, flaxseed meal, baking powder, and cinnamon.

2. In a separate bowl, combine mashed banana, almond milk, vanilla extract, and chopped walnuts.

3. Add the wet ingredients to the dry ingredients and mix until just combined.

4. Heat a non-stick pan over medium heat and ladle the batter onto the pan to form pancakes.

5. Cook until bubbles appear on the surface, then flip and cook the other side until golden brown.

6. Serve with a drizzle of maple syrup if desired. These vegan pancakes are a kidney-friendly treat.

Nutritional Information (per serving):

- Calories: 320

- Protein: 10g

- Carbohydrates: 45g

- Fiber: 8g

- Potassium: 350mg

- Phosphorus: 200mg

6. Berry Smoothie Bowl

Prep Time: 5 minutes

Cooking Time: 0 minutes

Serving Size: 1

Ingredients:

- 1 cup mixed berries (strawberries, blueberries, raspberries)

- 1/2 banana

- 1/2 cup unsweetened almond milk

- 1 tablespoon almond butter

- 2 tablespoons rolled oats

- Toppings: sliced banana, chia seeds, shredded coconut

Instructions:

1. In a blender, combine mixed berries, banana, almond milk, almond butter, and rolled oats. Blend until smooth.

2. Pour the smoothie into a bowl and arrange toppings like sliced banana, chia seeds, and shredded coconut.

3. Enjoy this nutrient-packed smoothie bowl, providing a delicious and kidney-friendly start to your day.

Nutritional Information (per serving):

- Calories: 280

- Protein: 8g

- Carbohydrates: 40g

- Fiber: 10g

- Potassium: 350mg

- Phosphorus: 180mg

7. Vegan Tofu Pancakes with Blueberry Compote

Prep Time: 15 minutes

Cooking Time: 15 minutes

Serving Size: 2

Ingredients:

- 1 cup all-purpose flour

- 1 tablespoon sugar

- 1 teaspoon baking powder

- 1/2 teaspoon baking soda

- 1/4 teaspoon salt

- 1 cup almond milk

- 1 tablespoon apple cider vinegar

- 1/2 teaspoon vanilla extract

- 1/2 cup silken tofu, blended until smooth

- Cooking spray

Blueberry Compote:

- 1 cup blueberries

- 1 tablespoon maple syrup

- 1 teaspoon lemon juice

Instructions:

1. In a bowl, whisk together flour, sugar, baking powder, baking soda, and salt.

2. In a separate bowl, mix almond milk, apple cider vinegar, vanilla extract, and blended silken tofu.

3. Combine the wet and dry ingredients until just mixed.

4. Heat a griddle or non-stick pan over medium heat. Lightly coat with cooking spray.

5. Pour 1/4 cup of batter for each pancake onto the griddle. Cook until bubbles appear, then flip and cook the other side.

6. For the blueberry compote, simmer blueberries, maple syrup, and lemon juice in a saucepan until berries burst.

7. Serve the pancakes topped with blueberry compote. This kidney-friendly breakfast is a delightful treat.

Nutritional Information (per serving):

- Calories: 320

- Protein: 8g

- Carbohydrates: 60g

- Fiber: 4g

- Potassium: 350mg

- Phosphorus: 180mg

8. Vegan Breakfast Burrito

Prep Time: 15 minutes

Cooking Time: 10 minutes

Serving Size: 1

Ingredients:

- 1 whole-grain tortilla

- 1/2 cup black beans, cooked and mashed

- 1/4 cup avocado, sliced

- 1/4 cup salsa

- 1/4 cup spinach, chopped

- 2 tablespoons nutritional yeast

- Salt and pepper to taste

Instructions:

1. Warm the tortilla in a dry skillet for 30 seconds on each side.

2. Spread mashed black beans down the center of the tortilla.

3. Layer with sliced avocado, salsa, chopped spinach, and nutritional yeast.

4. Season with salt and pepper to taste.

5. Fold the sides of the tortilla over the filling to form a burrito.

6. Serve warm, providing a protein-rich and kidney-friendly breakfast.

Nutritional Information (per serving):

- Calories: 320

- Protein: 12g

- Carbohydrates: 45g

- Fiber: 10g

- Potassium: 400mg

- Phosphorus: 220mg

9. Vegan Sweet Potato and Black Bean Hash

Prep Time: 15 minutes

Cooking Time: 20 minutes

Serving Size: 2

Ingredients:

- 2 medium sweet potatoes, peeled and diced

- 1 can (15 oz) black beans, drained and rinsed

- 1 bell pepper, diced

- 1/2 red onion, diced

- 2 tablespoons olive oil

- 1 teaspoon ground cumin

- 1/2 teaspoon smoked paprika

- Salt and pepper to taste

Instructions:

1. In a large skillet, heat olive oil over medium heat. Add diced sweet potatoes and cook until tender (about 15 minutes).

2. Add diced bell pepper and red onion to the skillet, cooking for an additional 5 minutes.

3. Stir in black beans, ground cumin, smoked paprika, salt, and pepper. Cook for another 5 minutes until well combined.

4. Serve warm, providing a hearty and kidney-friendly breakfast.

Nutritional Information (per serving):

- Calories: 330

- Protein: 10g

- Carbohydrates: 50g

- Fiber: 12g

- Potassium: 420mg

- Phosphorus: 180mg

10. Vegan Spinach and Mushroom Frittata

Prep Time: 15 minutes

Cooking Time: 25 minutes

Serving Size: 4

Ingredients:

- 1 cup chickpea flour

- 1 1/2 cups water

- 1 tablespoon nutritional yeast

- 1 teaspoon turmeric powder

- 1/2 teaspoon baking powder

- 1 tablespoon olive oil

- 1 onion, diced

- 2 cups spinach, chopped

- 1 cup mushrooms, sliced

- Salt and pepper to taste

Instructions:

1. Preheat the oven to 375°F (190°C).

2. In a blender, combine chickpea flour, water, nutritional yeast, turmeric powder, and baking powder. Blend until smooth.

3. In an oven-safe skillet, heat olive oil over medium heat. Add diced onion and cook until translucent.

4. Add chopped spinach and mushrooms to the skillet, cooking until spinach wilts and mushrooms are tender.

5. Pour the chickpea flour mixture over the vegetables in the skillet.

6. Transfer the skillet to the preheated oven and bake for 20-25 minutes until the frittata is set.

7. Slice into wedges and serve. This protein-rich frittata is a satisfying and kidney-friendly breakfast option.

Nutritional Information (per serving):

- Calories: 250

- Protein: 12g

- Carbohydrates: 30g

- Fiber: 7g

- Potassium: 320mg

- Phosphorus: 150mg

11. Vegan Chia Seed Pancakes with Mixed Berry Compote

Prep Time: 15 minutes

Cooking Time: 15 minutes

Serving Size: 2

Ingredients:

- 1 cup all-purpose flour

- 2 tablespoons chia seeds

- 1 tablespoon sugar

- 1 teaspoon baking powder

- 1/2 teaspoon baking soda

- 1/4 teaspoon salt

- 1 cup almond milk

- 1 tablespoon apple cider vinegar

- 1/2 teaspoon vanilla extract

- Cooking spray

Mixed Berry Compote:

- 1/2 cup strawberries, sliced

- 1/2 cup blueberries

- 1 tablespoon maple syrup

- 1 teaspoon lemon juice

Instructions:

1. In a bowl, whisk together flour, chia seeds, sugar, baking powder, baking soda, and salt.

2. In a separate bowl, mix almond milk, apple cider vinegar, and vanilla extract.

3. Combine the wet and dry ingredients until just mixed.

4. Heat a griddle or non-stick pan over medium heat. Lightly coat with cooking spray.

5. Pour 1/4 cup of batter for each pancake onto the griddle. Cook until bubbles appear, then flip and cook the other side.

6. For the mixed berry compote, simmer strawberries, blueberries, maple syrup, and lemon juice in a saucepan until berries burst.

7. Serve the pancakes topped with mixed berry compote. This delicious and kidney-friendly breakfast is perfect for a delightful morning.

Nutritional Information (per serving):

- Calories: 320

- Protein: 8g

- Carbohydrates: 60g

- Fiber: 5g

- Potassium: 330mg

- Phosphorus: 180mg

12. Vegan Tofu and Vegetable Breakfast Burrito

Prep Time: 15 minutes

Cooking Time: 10 minutes

Serving Size: 1

Ingredients:

- 1 whole-grain tortilla

- 1/2 cup extra-firm tofu, crumbled

- 1/4 cup black beans, cooked and mashed

- 1/4 cup avocado, sliced

- 1/4 cup salsa

- 1/4 cup bell peppers, diced

- 2 tablespoons nutritional yeast

- Salt and pepper to taste

Instructions:

1. Warm the tortilla in a dry skillet for 30 seconds on each side.

2. In a separate skillet, sauté crumbled tofu and diced bell peppers until tofu is lightly browned.

3. Spread mashed black beans down the center of the tortilla.

4. Layer with crumbled tofu, sliced avocado, salsa, and nutritional yeast.

5. Season with salt and pepper to taste.

6. Fold the sides of the tortilla over the filling to form a burrito.

7. Serve warm, providing a protein-rich and kidney-friendly breakfast.

Nutritional Information (per serving):

- Calories: 340

- Protein: 15g

- Carbohydrates: 45g

- Fiber: 10g

- Potassium: 420mg

- Phosphorus: 220mg

13. Vegan Quinoa Breakfast Bowl

Prep Time: 15 minutes

Cooking Time: 15 minutes

Serving Size: 2

Ingredients:

- 1 cup cooked quinoa

- 1/2 cup coconut milk

- 1 tablespoon maple syrup

- 1/4 cup almonds, chopped

- 1/4 cup dried cranberries

- 1/2 banana, sliced

- 1 tablespoon hemp seeds

Instructions:

1. In a saucepan, heat coconut milk over medium heat. Stir in cooked quinoa and maple syrup.

2. Cook for 5-7 minutes until the mixture is warmed through and slightly thickened.

3. Divide the quinoa mixture into bowls and top with chopped almonds, dried cranberries, sliced banana, and hemp seeds.

4. Drizzle with additional maple syrup if desired. This nutrient-rich and kidney-friendly breakfast bowl is a delicious start to your day.

Nutritional Information (per serving):

- Calories: 320

- Protein: 8g

- Carbohydrates: 50g

- Fiber: 7g

- Potassium: 380mg

- Phosphorus: 180mg

14. Vegan Chickpea Flour Crepes with Berry Compote

Prep Time: 15 minutes

Cooking Time: 20 minutes

Serving Size: 2

Ingredients: Crepes:

- 1 cup chickpea flour

- 1 1/2 cups water

- 1 tablespoon coconut oil, melted

- 1/2 teaspoon vanilla extract

- Pinch of salt

Berry Compote:

- 1 cup mixed berries (strawberries, blueberries, raspberries)

- 1 tablespoon maple syrup

- 1 teaspoon lemon juice

Instructions:

1. In a blender, combine chickpea flour, water, melted coconut oil, vanilla extract, and a pinch of salt. Blend until smooth.

2. Heat a non-stick skillet over medium heat. Pour a small amount of batter onto the skillet, swirling to spread evenly.

3. Cook each crepe for 2-3 minutes on each side, until lightly golden.

4. For the berry compote, simmer mixed berries, maple syrup, and lemon juice in a saucepan until berries burst.

5. Fill each crepe with the berry compote and fold into quarters. Serve warm, creating a delightful and kidney-friendly breakfast.

Nutritional Information (per serving):

- Calories: 280

- Protein: 8g

- Carbohydrates: 40g

- Fiber: 7g

- Potassium: 330mg

- Phosphorus: 150mg

15. Vegan Breakfast Quinoa Bowl with Almond Butter and Banana

Prep Time: 10 minutes

Cooking Time: 15 minutes

Serving Size: 1

Ingredients:

- 1/2 cup cooked quinoa

- 1/2 cup almond milk

- 1 tablespoon almond butter

- 1 banana, sliced

- 1 tablespoon chopped almonds

- 1 teaspoon maple syrup

Instructions:

1. In a saucepan, heat almond milk over medium heat. Stir in cooked quinoa until warmed through.

2. Transfer the quinoa to a bowl and top with almond butter, sliced banana, chopped almonds, and a drizzle of maple syrup.

3. Mix well and enjoy this protein-packed and kidney-friendly breakfast.

Nutritional Information (per serving):

- Calories: 290

- Protein: 8g

- Carbohydrates: 45g

- Fiber: 6g

- Potassium: 380mg

- Phosphorus: 180mg

16. Vegan Almond and Berry Breakfast Parfait

Prep Time: 10 minutes

Cooking Time: 0 minutes

Serving Size: 1

Ingredients:

- 1/2 cup almond yogurt

- 1/4 cup granola (low-phosphorus)

- 1/2 cup mixed berries (blueberries, strawberries, raspberries)

- 1 tablespoon sliced almonds

- Drizzle of agave syrup

Instructions:

1. In a glass or bowl, layer almond yogurt with granola, mixed berries, and sliced almonds.

2. Drizzle agave syrup over the top for added sweetness.

3. Enjoy this refreshing and kidney-friendly breakfast parfait.

Nutritional Information (per serving):

- Calories: 250

- Protein: 6g

- Carbohydrates: 35g

- Fiber: 8g

- Potassium: 300mg

- Phosphorus: 120mg

17. Vegan Chocolate Chia Seed Pudding

Prep Time: 10 minutes (plus overnight refrigeration)

Cooking Time: 0 minutes

Serving Size: 1

Ingredients:

- 2 tablespoons chia seeds

- 1 cup unsweetened almond milk

- 1 tablespoon cocoa powder

- 1 tablespoon maple syrup

- 1/2 teaspoon vanilla extract

Instructions:

1. In a bowl, mix chia seeds, almond milk, cocoa powder, maple syrup, and vanilla extract. Stir well and refrigerate overnight.

2. In the morning, give the chocolate chia pudding a good stir.

3. Enjoy this rich and kidney-friendly chocolate treat for breakfast.

Nutritional Information (per serving):

- Calories: 220

- Protein: 5g

- Carbohydrates: 30g

- Fiber: 10g

- Potassium: 280mg

- Phosphorus: 120mg

18. Vegan Blueberry and Almond Overnight Oats

Prep Time: 10 minutes (plus overnight refrigeration)

Cooking Time: 0 minutes

Serving Size: 1

Ingredients:

- 1/2 cup old-fashioned oats

- 1/2 cup unsweetened almond milk

- 1/4 cup blueberries

- 1 tablespoon almond butter

- 1 teaspoon maple syrup

- 1 tablespoon sliced almonds

Instructions:

1. In a jar, combine oats, almond milk, blueberries, almond butter, and maple syrup. Stir well and refrigerate overnight.

2. In the morning, give the overnight oats a good stir.

3. Top with sliced almonds and enjoy this convenient and kidney-friendly breakfast.

Nutritional Information (per serving):

- Calories: 280

- Protein: 7g

- Carbohydrates: 40g

- Fiber: 8g

- Potassium: 300mg

- Phosphorus: 150mg

19. Vegan Spinach and Mushroom Breakfast Wrap

Prep Time: 10 minutes

Cooking Time: 10 minutes

Serving Size: 1

Ingredients:

- 1 whole-grain tortilla

- 1/2 cup extra-firm tofu, crumbled

- 1/4 cup black beans, cooked and mashed

- 1/4 cup avocado, sliced

- 1/4 cup salsa

- 1/4 cup spinach, chopped

- 2 tablespoons nutritional yeast

- Salt and pepper to taste

Instructions:

1. Warm the tortilla in a dry skillet for 30 seconds on each side.

2. In a separate skillet, sauté crumbled tofu and chopped spinach until tofu is lightly browned.

3. Spread mashed black beans down the center of the tortilla.

4. Layer with crumbled tofu, sliced avocado, salsa, and nutritional yeast.

5. Season with salt and pepper to taste.

6. Fold the sides of the tortilla over the filling to form a wrap.

7. Serve warm, providing a protein-rich and kidney-friendly breakfast.

Nutritional Information (per serving):

- Calories: 340

- Protein: 15g

- Carbohydrates: 45g

- Fiber: 10g

- Potassium: 420mg

- Phosphorus: 220mg

20. Vegan Peanut Butter and Banana Toast

Prep Time: 5 minutes

Cooking Time: 5 minutes

Serving Size: 1

Ingredients:

- 1 slice whole-grain bread

- 2 tablespoons peanut butter

- 1 banana, sliced

- Drizzle of agave syrup

Instructions:

1. Toast the whole-grain bread to your desired level of crispiness.

2. Spread peanut butter evenly over the toasted bread.

3. Arrange sliced banana on top of the peanut butter.

4. Drizzle with agave syrup for added sweetness.

5. Enjoy this quick and kidney-friendly breakfast toast.

Nutritional Information (per serving):

- Calories: 290

- Protein: 7g

- Carbohydrates: 40g

- Fiber: 7g

- Potassium: 380mg

- Phosphorus: 180mg

LUNCH RECIPES

1. Vegan Lentil and Vegetable Stew

Prep Time: 15 minutes

Cooking Time: 40 minutes

Serving Size: 4

Ingredients:

- 1 cup green lentils, rinsed

- 4 cups vegetable broth

- 1 onion, chopped

- 2 carrots, diced

- 2 celery stalks, chopped

- 3 cloves garlic, minced

- 1 can (15 oz) diced tomatoes

- 1 teaspoon cumin

- 1 teaspoon paprika

- Salt and pepper to taste

- Fresh parsley for garnish

Instructions:

1. In a large pot, combine lentils, vegetable broth, onion, carrots, celery, and garlic.

2. Bring to a boil, then reduce heat and simmer for 30-40 minutes until lentils are tender.

3. Add diced tomatoes, cumin, paprika, salt, and pepper. Cook for an additional 10 minutes.

4. Garnish with fresh parsley before serving. This hearty stew is a nutritious and kidney-friendly lunch option.

Nutritional Information (per serving):

- Calories: 250

- Protein: 15g

- Carbohydrates: 45g

- Fiber: 15g

- Potassium: 600mg

- Phosphorus: 230mg

2. Vegan Quinoa Salad with Chickpeas and Vegetables

Prep Time: 20 minutes

Cooking Time: 15 minutes

Serving Size: 3

Ingredients:

- 1 cup quinoa, cooked

- 1 can (15 oz) chickpeas, drained and rinsed

- 1 cucumber, diced

- 1 bell pepper, chopped

- 1 cup cherry tomatoes, halved

- 1/4 cup red onion, finely chopped

- 1/4 cup fresh parsley, chopped

Dressing:

- 2 tablespoons olive oil

- 1 tablespoon lemon juice

- 1 teaspoon Dijon mustard

- Salt and pepper to taste

Instructions:

1. In a large bowl, combine cooked quinoa, chickpeas, cucumber, bell pepper, cherry tomatoes, red onion, and fresh parsley.

2. In a small bowl, whisk together olive oil, lemon juice, Dijon mustard, salt, and pepper to make the dressing.

3. Pour the dressing over the salad and toss to combine.

4. Chill in the refrigerator for at least 30 minutes before serving. This refreshing quinoa salad is kidney-friendly and packed with nutrients.

Nutritional Information (per serving):

- Calories: 320

- Protein: 14g

- Carbohydrates: 50g

- Fiber: 10g

- Potassium: 450mg

- Phosphorus: 220mg

3. Vegan Chickpea and Spinach Curry

Prep Time: 15 minutes

Cooking Time: 25 minutes

Serving Size: 2

Ingredients:

- 1 can (15 oz) chickpeas, drained and rinsed

- 1 onion, finely chopped

- 2 cloves garlic, minced

- 1 teaspoon ginger, grated

- 1 can (14 oz) coconut milk

- 1 can (14 oz) diced tomatoes

- 2 cups fresh spinach

- 1 tablespoon curry powder

- 1 teaspoon turmeric

- Salt and pepper to taste

- Cooked brown rice for serving

Instructions:

1. In a large skillet, sauté chopped onion, garlic, and ginger until softened.

2. Add chickpeas, coconut milk, diced tomatoes, curry powder, turmeric, salt, and pepper. Simmer for 20 minutes.

3. Stir in fresh spinach and cook until wilted.

4. Serve over cooked brown rice. This flavorful chickpea and spinach curry provide a kidney-friendly and satisfying lunch.

Nutritional Information (per serving):

- Calories: 400

- Protein: 15g

- Carbohydrates: 50g

- Fiber: 12g

- Potassium: 550mg

- Phosphorus: 250mg

4. Vegan Mediterranean Quinoa Bowl

Prep Time: 15 minutes

Cooking Time: 15 minutes

Serving Size: 3

Ingredients:

- 1 cup quinoa, cooked

- 1 cup cherry tomatoes, halved

- 1 cucumber, diced

- 1/2 cup Kalamata olives, sliced

- 1/4 cup red onion, finely chopped

- 1/4 cup fresh parsley, chopped

Dressing:

- 3 tablespoons olive oil

- 1 tablespoon balsamic vinegar

- 1 teaspoon dried oregano

- Salt and pepper to taste

Instructions:

1. In a large bowl, combine cooked quinoa, cherry tomatoes, cucumber, Kalamata olives, red onion, and fresh parsley.

2. In a small bowl, whisk together olive oil, balsamic vinegar, dried oregano, salt, and pepper to make the dressing.

3. Pour the dressing over the quinoa bowl and toss to combine.

4. Chill in the refrigerator for at least 30 minutes before serving. This Mediterranean-inspired quinoa bowl is kidney-friendly and bursting with flavors.

Nutritional Information (per serving):

- Calories: 320

- Protein: 10g

- Carbohydrates: 45g

- Fiber: 8g

- Potassium: 400mg

- Phosphorus: 200mg

5. Vegan Sweet Potato and Black Bean Burrito Bowl

Prep Time: 20 minutes

Cooking Time: 25 minutes

Serving Size: 2

Ingredients:

- 1 cup brown rice, cooked

- 1 sweet potato, peeled and diced

- 1 can (15 oz) black beans, drained and rinsed

- 1/2 cup corn kernels

- 1/2 cup cherry tomatoes, halved

- 1/4 cup red onion, finely chopped

- 1/4 cup fresh cilantro, chopped

Avocado Lime Dressing:

- 1 avocado, mashed

- 1 lime, juiced

- 2 tablespoons olive oil

- Salt and pepper to taste

Instructions:

1. Roast sweet potato cubes in the oven until tender.

2. In a bowl, assemble cooked brown rice, roasted sweet potato, black beans, corn, cherry tomatoes, red onion, and fresh cilantro.

3. In a separate bowl, mix mashed avocado, lime juice, olive oil, salt, and pepper to make the dressing.

4. Drizzle the avocado lime dressing over the burrito bowl before serving. This nutrient-rich and kidney-friendly lunch option is both delicious and satisfying.

Nutritional Information (per serving):

- Calories: 380

- Protein: 12g

- Carbohydrates: 60g

- Fiber: 10g

- Potassium: 500mg

- Phosphorus: 220mg

6. Vegan Roasted Vegetable and Quinoa Salad

Prep Time: 20 minutes

Cooking Time: 25 minutes

Serving Size: 3

Ingredients:

- 1 cup quinoa, cooked

- 1 zucchini, sliced

- 1 bell pepper, sliced

- 1 red onion, sliced

- 1 cup cherry tomatoes, halved

- 2 tablespoons olive oil

- 1 teaspoon dried thyme

- Salt and pepper to taste

- 1/4 cup fresh basil, chopped

Lemon Tahini Dressing:

- 3 tablespoons tahini

- 1 lemon, juiced

- 2 tablespoons water

- 1 clove garlic, minced

- Salt and pepper to taste

Instructions:

1. Preheat the oven to 400°F (200°C).

2. Toss sliced zucchini, bell pepper, red onion, and cherry tomatoes with olive oil, dried thyme, salt, and pepper. Roast in the oven for 20-25 minutes until vegetables are golden brown.

3. In a large bowl, combine cooked quinoa, roasted vegetables, and fresh basil.

4. In a small bowl, whisk together tahini, lemon juice, water, minced garlic, salt, and pepper to make the dressing.

5. Drizzle the lemon tahini dressing over the salad before serving. This vibrant and kidney-friendly roasted vegetable and quinoa salad is a delightful lunch option.

Nutritional Information (per serving):

- Calories: 350

- Protein: 10g

- Carbohydrates: 45g

- Fiber: 8g

- Potassium: 450mg

- Phosphorus: 220mg

7. Vegan Black Bean and Corn Quesadillas

Prep Time: 15 minutes

Cooking Time: 15 minutes

Serving Size: 2

Ingredients:

- 4 whole-grain tortillas

- 1 can (15 oz) black beans, drained and rinsed

- 1 cup corn kernels

- 1/2 cup red onion, finely chopped

- 1/2 cup bell pepper, diced

- 1 teaspoon cumin

- 1/2 teaspoon chili powder

- Salt and pepper to taste

- 1 cup vegan cheese, shredded

- Fresh cilantro for garnish

Instructions:

1. In a bowl, mix black beans, corn, red onion, bell pepper, cumin, chili powder, salt, and pepper.

2. Place a tortilla on a flat surface and spread a portion of the bean mixture on half of the tortilla.

3. Sprinkle vegan cheese over the bean mixture and fold the tortilla in half.

4. Repeat with the remaining tortillas.

5. Heat a non-stick skillet over medium heat. Cook each quesadilla for 3-4 minutes on each side until golden brown.

6. Garnish with fresh cilantro before serving. These black bean and corn quesadillas are a kidney-friendly and flavorful lunch.

Nutritional Information (per serving):

- Calories: 380

- Protein: 15g

- Carbohydrates: 55g

- Fiber: 12g

- Potassium: 500mg

- Phosphorus: 250mg

8. Vegan Eggplant and Tomato Pasta

Prep Time: 20 minutes

Cooking Time: 25 minutes

Serving Size: 3

Ingredients:

- 8 oz whole-grain pasta, cooked

- 1 large eggplant, diced

- 1 cup cherry tomatoes, halved

- 3 cloves garlic, minced

- 2 tablespoons olive oil

- 1 teaspoon dried oregano

- 1/2 teaspoon red pepper flakes

- Salt and pepper to taste

- Fresh basil for garnish

Instructions:

1. In a large skillet, sauté diced eggplant, cherry tomatoes, and minced garlic in olive oil until eggplant is golden brown.

2. Add dried oregano, red pepper flakes, salt, and pepper. Cook for an additional 5 minutes.

3. Toss cooked pasta into the skillet and mix well.

4. Garnish with fresh basil before serving. This eggplant and tomato pasta is a kidney-friendly and satisfying lunch option.

Nutritional Information (per serving):

- Calories: 350

- Protein: 10g

- Carbohydrates: 55g

- Fiber: 12g

- Potassium: 450mg

- Phosphorus: 200mg

9. Vegan Butternut Squash and Kale Salad

Prep Time: 15 minutes

Cooking Time: 25 minutes

Serving Size: 2

Ingredients:

- 1/2 butternut squash, peeled and diced

- 4 cups kale, stems removed and chopped

- 1/4 cup walnuts, chopped

- 1/4 cup dried cranberries

- 2 tablespoons olive oil

- 1 tablespoon balsamic vinegar

- 1 teaspoon maple syrup

- Salt and pepper to taste

Instructions:

1. Roast diced butternut squash in the oven until tender.

2. In a large bowl, combine chopped kale, roasted butternut squash, chopped walnuts, and dried cranberries.

3. In a small bowl, whisk together olive oil, balsamic vinegar, maple syrup, salt, and pepper to make the dressing.

4. Pour the dressing over the salad and toss to combine. This butternut squash and kale salad is a nutritious and kidney-friendly lunch.

Nutritional Information (per serving):

- Calories: 300

- Protein: 8g

- Carbohydrates: 40g

- Fiber: 8g

- Potassium: 500mg

- Phosphorus: 180mg

10. Vegan Cauliflower and Chickpea Curry

Prep Time: 20 minutes

Cooking Time: 25 minutes

Serving Size: 3

Ingredients:

- 1 cauliflower, cut into florets

- 1 can (15 oz) chickpeas, drained and rinsed

- 1 onion, finely chopped

- 2 cloves garlic, minced

- 1 can (14 oz) coconut milk

- 2 tablespoons curry powder

- 1 teaspoon turmeric

- Salt and pepper to taste

- Fresh cilantro for garnish

- Cooked brown rice for serving

Instructions:

1. In a large pot, sauté chopped onion and minced garlic until softened.

2. Add cauliflower florets, chickpeas, coconut milk, curry powder, turmeric, salt, and pepper. Simmer for 20 minutes.

3. Serve over cooked brown rice and garnish with fresh cilantro. This cauliflower and chickpea curry is a flavorful and kidney-friendly lunch option.

Nutritional Information (per serving):

- Calories: 380

- Protein: 12g

- Carbohydrates: 50g

- Fiber: 12g

- Potassium: 550mg

- Phosphorus: 250mg

11. Vegan Spinach and Mushroom Stuffed Bell Peppers

Prep Time: 20 minutes

Cooking Time: 30 minutes

Serving Size: 2

Ingredients:

- 2 bell peppers, halved and seeds removed

- 2 cups spinach, chopped

- 1 cup mushrooms, diced

- 1 cup cooked quinoa

- 1/4 cup nutritional yeast

- 2 cloves garlic, minced

- 1 teaspoon olive oil

- Salt and pepper to taste

- Marinara sauce for serving

Instructions:

1. Preheat the oven to 375°F (190°C).

2. In a skillet, sauté chopped spinach, diced mushrooms, and minced garlic in olive oil until spinach is wilted.

3. In a bowl, mix cooked quinoa, nutritional yeast, sautéed spinach and mushrooms, salt, and pepper.

4. Stuff each bell pepper half with the quinoa mixture.

5. Place stuffed bell peppers in a baking dish and bake for 25-30 minutes until peppers are tender.

6. Serve with marinara sauce. These spinach and mushroom stuffed bell peppers are a kidney-friendly and satisfying lunch option.

Nutritional Information (per serving):

- Calories: 320

- Protein: 10g

- Carbohydrates: 45g

- Fiber: 10g

- Potassium: 400mg

- Phosphorus: 180mg

12. Vegan Sweet and Spicy Tofu Stir-Fry

Prep Time: 20 minutes

Cooking Time: 15 minutes

Serving Size: 3

Ingredients:

- 1 block extra-firm tofu, cubed

- 2 cups broccoli florets

- 1 bell pepper, sliced

- 1 carrot, julienned

- 1/2 cup snow peas

- 3 tablespoons soy sauce

- 2 tablespoons maple syrup

- 1 tablespoon rice vinegar

- 1 tablespoon cornstarch

- 1 teaspoon sesame oil

- 1 teaspoon ginger, grated

- 2 cloves garlic, minced

- Cooked brown rice for serving

Instructions:

1. Press tofu to remove excess water, then cube.

2. In a wok or large skillet, stir-fry tofu until golden brown. Remove from the wok and set aside.

3. In the same wok, stir-fry broccoli, bell pepper, carrot, and snow peas until vegetables are tender-crisp.

4. In a bowl, whisk together soy sauce, maple syrup, rice vinegar, cornstarch, sesame oil, grated ginger, and minced garlic.

5. Pour the sauce over the vegetables and add the cooked tofu. Stir-fry for an additional 3-5 minutes.

6. Serve over cooked brown rice. This sweet and spicy tofu stir-fry is a flavorful and kidney-friendly lunch option.

Nutritional Information (per serving):

- Calories: 350

- Protein: 15g

- Carbohydrates: 50g

- Fiber: 8g

- Potassium: 500mg

- Phosphorus: 220mg

13. Vegan Zucchini Noodles with Pesto

Prep Time: 15 minutes

Cooking Time: 0 minutes

Serving Size: 2

Ingredients:

- 2 large zucchini, spiralized

- 1 cup cherry tomatoes, halved

- 1/4 cup pine nuts, toasted

- 1/4 cup nutritional yeast

- 2 tablespoons olive oil

- 1 clove garlic, minced

- 1 cup fresh basil leaves

- Salt and pepper to taste

Instructions:

1. Spiralize zucchini to create noodles.

2. In a blender, combine cherry tomatoes, toasted pine nuts, nutritional yeast, olive oil, minced garlic, fresh basil, salt, and pepper. Blend until smooth to make the pesto.

3. Toss zucchini noodles with the pesto until well-coated.

4. Serve chilled or at room temperature. These zucchini noodles with pesto are a light and kidney-friendly lunch option.

Nutritional Information (per serving):

- Calories: 280

- Protein: 8g

- Carbohydrates: 30g

- Fiber: 7g

- Potassium: 400mg

- Phosphorus: 150mg

14. Vegan Lentil and Vegetable Stir-Fry

Prep Time: 20 minutes

Cooking Time: 15 minutes

Serving Size: 3

Ingredients:

- 1 cup green lentils, cooked

- 2 cups broccoli florets

- 1 bell pepper, sliced

- 1 carrot, julienned

- 1/2 cup snap peas

- 3 tablespoons soy sauce

- 2 tablespoons hoisin sauce

- 1 tablespoon sesame oil

- 1 teaspoon ginger, grated

- 2 cloves garlic, minced

- Cooked quinoa for serving

Instructions:

1. In a wok or large skillet, stir-fry cooked green lentils, broccoli, bell pepper, carrot, and snap peas until vegetables are tender-crisp.

2. In a bowl, whisk together soy sauce, hoisin sauce, sesame oil, grated ginger, and minced garlic.

3. Pour the sauce over the lentil and vegetable mixture. Stir-fry for an additional 3-5 minutes.

4. Serve over cooked quinoa. This lentil and vegetable stir-fry is a protein-packed and kidney-friendly lunch option.

Nutritional Information (per serving):

- Calories: 380

- Protein: 18g

- Carbohydrates: 50g

- Fiber: 12g

- Potassium: 550mg

- Phosphorus: 250mg

15. Vegan Stuffed Bell Peppers with Quinoa and Black Beans

Prep Time: 20 minutes

Cooking Time: 30 minutes

Serving Size: 2

Ingredients:

- 2 bell peppers, halved and seeds removed

- 1 cup cooked quinoa

- 1 can (15 oz) black beans, drained and rinsed

- 1 cup corn kernels

- 1/2 cup salsa

- 1 teaspoon cumin

- 1/2 teaspoon chili powder

- Salt and pepper to taste

- Vegan cheese for topping

Instructions:

1. Preheat the oven to 375°F (190°C).

2. In a bowl, mix cooked quinoa, black beans, corn, salsa, cumin, chili powder, salt, and pepper.

3. Stuff each bell pepper half with the quinoa mixture.

4. Top with vegan cheese and bake for 25-30 minutes until peppers are tender.

5. Serve with additional salsa if desired. These stuffed bell peppers with quinoa and black beans are a kidney-friendly and satisfying lunch option.

Nutritional Information (per serving):

- Calories: 350

- Protein: 14g

- Carbohydrates: 55g

- Fiber: 12g

- Potassium: 500mg

- Phosphorus: 220mg

16. Vegan Chickpea and Vegetable Stir-Fry

Prep Time: 20 minutes

Cooking Time: 15 minutes

Serving Size: 3

Ingredients:

- 1 can (15 oz) chickpeas, drained and rinsed

- 2 cups broccoli florets

- 1 bell pepper, sliced

- 1 carrot, julienned

- 1/2 cup snap peas

- 3 tablespoons soy sauce

- 2 tablespoons hoisin sauce

- 1 tablespoon sesame oil

- 1 teaspoon ginger, grated

- 2 cloves garlic, minced

- Cooked brown rice for serving

Instructions:

1. In a wok or large skillet, stir-fry chickpeas, broccoli, bell pepper, carrot, and snap peas until vegetables are tender-crisp.

2. In a bowl, whisk together soy sauce, hoisin sauce, sesame oil, grated ginger, and minced garlic.

3. Pour the sauce over the chickpea and vegetable mixture. Stir-fry for an additional 3-5 minutes.

4. Serve over cooked brown rice. This chickpea and vegetable stir-fry is a protein-rich and kidney-friendly lunch option.

Nutritional Information (per serving):

- Calories: 360

- Protein: 15g

- Carbohydrates: 50g

- Fiber: 10g

- Potassium: 450mg

- Phosphorus: 220mg

17. Vegan Mediterranean Chickpea Salad

Prep Time: 15 minutes

Cooking Time: 0 minutes

Serving Size: 2

Ingredients:

- 1 can (15 oz) chickpeas, drained and rinsed

- 1 cucumber, diced

- 1 cup cherry tomatoes, halved

- 1/4 cup red onion, finely chopped

- 1/4 cup Kalamata olives, sliced

- 1/4 cup fresh parsley, chopped

Dressing:

- 3 tablespoons olive oil

- 1 tablespoon red wine vinegar

- 1 teaspoon dried oregano

- Salt and pepper to taste

Instructions:

1. In a large bowl, combine chickpeas, cucumber, cherry tomatoes, red onion, Kalamata olives, and fresh parsley.

2. In a small bowl, whisk together olive oil, red wine vinegar, dried oregano, salt, and pepper to make the dressing.

3. Pour the dressing over the salad and toss to combine.

4. Chill in the refrigerator for at least 30 minutes before serving. This Mediterranean chickpea salad is a refreshing and kidney-friendly lunch option.

Nutritional Information (per serving):

- Calories: 320

- Protein: 12g

- Carbohydrates: 45g

- Fiber: 12g

- Potassium: 500mg

- Phosphorus: 220mg

18. Vegan Avocado and Chickpea Wrap

Prep Time: 15 minutes

Cooking Time: 0 minutes

Serving Size: 1

Ingredients:

- 1 whole-grain tortilla

- 1/2 avocado, mashed

- 1/2 cup chickpeas, mashed

- 1/4 cup cucumber, diced

- 1/4 cup tomato, diced

- 2 tablespoons red onion, finely chopped

- 1 tablespoon fresh cilantro, chopped

- Juice of half a lime

- Salt and pepper to taste

Instructions:

1. In a bowl, combine mashed avocado, mashed chickpeas, cucumber, tomato, red onion, fresh cilantro, lime juice, salt, and pepper.

2. Warm the tortilla in a dry skillet for 30 seconds on each side.

3. Spread the avocado and chickpea mixture down the center of the tortilla.

4. Fold the sides of the tortilla over the filling to form a wrap.

5. Serve immediately. This avocado and chickpea wrap is a quick and kidney-friendly lunch option.

Nutritional Information (per serving):

- Calories: 380

- Protein: 10g

- Carbohydrates: 50g

- Fiber: 12g

- Potassium: 480mg

- Phosphorus: 220mg

19. Vegan Roasted Red Pepper and Hummus Sandwich

Prep Time: 10 minutes

Cooking Time: 0 minutes

Serving Size: 1

Ingredients:

- 2 slices whole-grain bread

- 1/4 cup hummus

- 1/2 cup roasted red peppers, sliced

- 1/4 cup cucumber, thinly sliced

- 1/4 cup baby spinach

- 1 tablespoon pumpkin seeds

- Sprinkle of black pepper

Instructions:

1. Spread hummus evenly on both slices of whole-grain bread.

2. Layer roasted red peppers, cucumber, and baby spinach on one slice of bread.

3. Sprinkle pumpkin seeds and black pepper over the vegetables.

4. Top with the second slice of bread to create a sandwich.

5. Slice in half and serve immediately. This roasted red pepper
   and hummus sandwich is a flavorful and kidney-friendly
   lunch option.

Nutritional Information (per serving):

- Calories: 320

- Protein: 12g

- Carbohydrates: 40g

- Fiber: 8g

- Potassium: 450mg

- Phosphorus: 180mg

20. Vegan Broccoli and Almond Stir-Fry

Prep Time: 15 minutes

Cooking Time: 15 minutes

Serving Size: 3

Ingredients:

- 2 cups broccoli florets

- 1 cup sliced mushrooms

- 1/2 cup sliced almonds

- 3 tablespoons soy sauce

- 2 tablespoons rice vinegar

- 1 tablespoon maple syrup

- 1 tablespoon cornstarch

- 1 teaspoon sesame oil

- 1 teaspoon ginger, grated

- 2 cloves garlic, minced

- Cooked brown rice for serving

Instructions:

1. In a wok or large skillet, stir-fry broccoli, mushrooms, and sliced almonds until vegetables are tender-crisp.

2. In a bowl, whisk together soy sauce, rice vinegar, maple syrup, cornstarch, sesame oil, grated ginger, and minced garlic.

3. Pour the sauce over the broccoli and almond mixture. Stir-fry for an additional 3-5 minutes.

4. Serve over cooked brown rice. This broccoli and almond stir-fry is a nutrient-packed and kidney-friendly lunch option.

Nutritional Information (per serving):

- Calories: 350

- Protein: 15g

- Carbohydrates: 45g

- Fiber: 10g

- Potassium: 500mg

- Phosphorus: 220mg

DINNER RECIPES

1. Vegan Chickpea and Vegetable Curry

Prep Time: 20 minutes

Cooking Time: 25 minutes

Serving Size: 4

Ingredients:

- 2 cans (15 oz each) chickpeas, drained and rinsed

- 1 eggplant, diced

- 1 bell pepper, chopped

- 1 zucchini, sliced

- 1 onion, finely chopped

- 2 cloves garlic, minced

- 1 can (14 oz) coconut milk

- 1 can (14 oz) diced tomatoes

- 2 tablespoons curry powder

- 1 teaspoon turmeric

- Salt and pepper to taste

- Fresh cilantro for garnish

- Cooked brown rice for serving

Instructions:

1. In a large pot, sauté chopped onion and minced garlic until softened.

2. Add chickpeas, diced eggplant, chopped bell pepper, sliced zucchini, coconut milk, diced tomatoes, curry powder, turmeric, salt, and pepper. Simmer for 20 minutes.

3. Serve over cooked brown rice and garnish with fresh cilantro. This flavorful chickpea and vegetable curry is a hearty and kidney-friendly dinner option.

Nutritional Information (per serving):

- Calories: 400

- Protein: 15g

- Carbohydrates: 55g

- Fiber: 12g

- Potassium: 550mg

- Phosphorus: 250mg

2. Vegan Lentil and Mushroom Stuffed Peppers

Prep Time: 20 minutes

Cooking Time: 30 minutes

Serving Size: 3

Ingredients:

- 1 cup green lentils, cooked

- 1 cup mushrooms, finely chopped

- 1 cup cooked quinoa

- 1/2 cup tomato sauce

- 1/4 cup red onion, finely chopped

- 2 cloves garlic, minced

- 1 teaspoon dried oregano

- 1/2 teaspoon red pepper flakes

- Salt and pepper to taste

- 3 bell peppers, halved and seeds removed

- Vegan cheese for topping

Instructions:

1. Preheat the oven to 375°F (190°C).

2. In a bowl, mix cooked green lentils, chopped mushrooms, cooked quinoa, tomato sauce, red onion, minced garlic, dried oregano, red pepper flakes, salt, and pepper.

3. Stuff each bell pepper half with the lentil and mushroom mixture.

4. Top with vegan cheese and bake for 25-30 minutes until peppers are tender.

5. Serve with additional tomato sauce if desired. These lentil and mushroom stuffed peppers are a kidney-friendly and satisfying dinner option.

Nutritional Information (per serving):

- Calories: 350

- Protein: 14g

- Carbohydrates: 50g

- Fiber: 12g

- Potassium: 500mg

- Phosphorus: 220mg

3. Vegan Quinoa and Vegetable Stir-Fry

Prep Time: 20 minutes

Cooking Time: 15 minutes

Serving Size: 4

Ingredients:

- 2 cups quinoa, cooked

- 1 cup broccoli florets

- 1 bell pepper, sliced

- 1 carrot, julienned

- 1/2 cup snap peas

- 1/4 cup soy sauce

- 2 tablespoons hoisin sauce

- 1 tablespoon sesame oil

- 1 teaspoon ginger, grated

- 2 cloves garlic, minced

- 1 tablespoon olive oil

Instructions:

1. In a wok or large skillet, stir-fry broccoli, bell pepper, carrot, and snap peas in olive oil until vegetables are tender-crisp.

2. Add cooked quinoa to the wok and stir to combine.

3. In a bowl, whisk together soy sauce, hoisin sauce, sesame oil, grated ginger, and minced garlic.

4. Pour the sauce over the quinoa and vegetable mixture. Stir-fry for an additional 3-5 minutes.

5. Serve immediately. This quinoa and vegetable stir-fry is a protein-packed and kidney-friendly dinner option.

Nutritional Information (per serving):

- Calories: 380

- Protein: 15g

- Carbohydrates: 50g

- Fiber: 10g

- Potassium: 450mg

- Phosphorus: 220mg

4. Vegan Spaghetti with Lentil Bolognese

Prep Time: 20 minutes

Cooking Time: 30 minutes

Serving Size: 4

Ingredients:

- 1 cup green lentils, cooked

- 2 cups whole-grain spaghetti, cooked

- 1 can (14 oz) crushed tomatoes

- 1 onion, finely chopped

- 2 cloves garlic, minced

- 1 carrot, grated

- 1 celery stalk, finely chopped

- 1 teaspoon dried oregano

- 1/2 teaspoon red pepper flakes

- Salt and pepper to taste

- Fresh basil for garnish

Instructions:

1. In a large skillet, sauté chopped onion and minced garlic until softened.

2. Add cooked green lentils, grated carrot, chopped celery, crushed tomatoes, dried oregano, red pepper flakes, salt, and pepper. Simmer for 20 minutes.

3. Serve the lentil Bolognese over cooked whole-grain spaghetti.

4. Garnish with fresh basil before serving. This hearty lentil Bolognese is a kidney-friendly and comforting dinner option.

Nutritional Information (per serving):

- Calories: 400

- Protein: 18g

- Carbohydrates: 60g

- Fiber: 15g

- Potassium: 550mg

- Phosphorus: 250mg

5. Vegan Sweet Potato and Black Bean Chili

Prep Time: 20 minutes

Cooking Time: 30 minutes

Serving Size: 4

Ingredients:

- 2 sweet potatoes, peeled and diced

- 1 can (15 oz) black beans, drained and rinsed

- 1 can (14 oz) diced tomatoes

- 1 onion, finely chopped

- 2 cloves garlic, minced

- 1 tablespoon chili powder

- 1 teaspoon cumin

- 1/2 teaspoon smoked paprika

- Salt and pepper to taste

- Fresh cilantro for garnish

- Vegan sour cream for serving

Instructions:

1. In a large pot, sauté chopped onion and minced garlic until softened.

2. Add diced sweet potatoes, black beans, diced tomatoes, chili powder, cumin, smoked paprika, salt, and pepper. Simmer for 25 minutes.

3. Serve the sweet potato and black bean chili hot, garnished with fresh cilantro and a dollop of vegan sour cream. This chili is a kidney-friendly and flavorful dinner option.

Nutritional Information (per serving):

- Calories: 350

- Protein: 12g

- Carbohydrates: 55g

- Fiber: 15g

- Potassium: 500mg

- Phosphorus: 220mg

6. Vegan Cauliflower and Chickpea Curry

Prep Time: 20 minutes

Cooking Time: 25 minutes

Serving Size: 4

Ingredients:

- 1 cauliflower, cut into florets

- 1 can (15 oz) chickpeas, drained and rinsed

- 1 onion, finely chopped

- 2 cloves garlic, minced

- 1 can (14 oz) coconut milk

- 2 tablespoons curry powder

- 1 teaspoon turmeric

- Salt and pepper to taste

- Fresh cilantro for garnish

- Cooked brown rice for serving

Instructions:

1. In a large pot, sauté chopped onion and minced garlic until softened.

2. Add cauliflower florets, chickpeas, coconut milk, curry powder, turmeric, salt, and pepper. Simmer for 20 minutes.

3. Serve over cooked brown rice and garnish with fresh cilantro. This cauliflower and chickpea curry is a flavorful and kidney-friendly dinner option.

Nutritional Information (per serving):

- Calories: 380

- Protein: 15g

- Carbohydrates: 50g

- Fiber: 12g

- Potassium: 550mg

- Phosphorus: 250mg

7. Vegan Stuffed Portobello Mushrooms

Prep Time: 20 minutes

Cooking Time: 25 minutes

Serving Size: 2

Ingredients:

- 4 large portobello mushrooms, stems removed

- 1 cup quinoa, cooked

- 1 cup spinach, chopped

- 1/4 cup sun-dried tomatoes, chopped

- 2 cloves garlic, minced

- 1/4 cup nutritional yeast

- 1 tablespoon olive oil

- Salt and pepper to taste

- Vegan Parmesan for topping

Instructions:

1. Preheat the oven to 375°F (190°C).

2. In a skillet, sauté chopped spinach, minced garlic, and sun-dried tomatoes in olive oil until spinach is wilted.

3. In a bowl, mix cooked quinoa, sautéed spinach mixture, nutritional yeast, salt, and pepper.

4. Stuff each portobello mushroom with the quinoa mixture and place on a baking sheet.

5. Bake for 20-25 minutes until mushrooms are tender.

6. Top with vegan Parmesan before serving. These stuffed portobello mushrooms are a kidney-friendly and savory dinner option.

Nutritional Information (per serving):

- Calories: 320

- Protein: 12g

- Carbohydrates: 45g

- Fiber: 10g

- Potassium: 450mg

- Phosphorus: 180mg

8. Vegan Mediterranean Couscous Salad

Prep Time: 15 minutes

Cooking Time: 10 minutes

Serving Size: 3

Ingredients:

- 1 cup whole-wheat couscous, cooked

- 1 cucumber, diced

- 1 cup cherry tomatoes, halved

- 1/4 cup Kalamata olives, sliced

- 1/4 cup red onion, finely chopped

- 1/4 cup fresh parsley, chopped

- 2 tablespoons olive oil

- 1 tablespoon red wine vinegar

- 1 teaspoon dried oregano

- Salt and pepper to taste

Instructions:

1. In a large bowl, combine cooked whole-wheat couscous, diced cucumber, halved cherry tomatoes, sliced Kalamata olives, chopped red onion, and fresh parsley.

2. In a small bowl, whisk together olive oil, red wine vinegar, dried oregano, salt, and pepper to make the dressing.

3. Pour the dressing over the salad and toss to combine.

4. Chill in the refrigerator for at least 30 minutes before serving. This Mediterranean couscous salad is a refreshing and kidney-friendly dinner option.

Nutritional Information (per serving):

- Calories: 300

- Protein: 10g

- Carbohydrates: 50g

- Fiber: 8g

- Potassium: 500mg

- Phosphorus: 200mg

9. Vegan Black Bean and Quinoa Stuffed Bell Peppers

Prep Time: 20 minutes

Cooking Time: 30 minutes

Serving Size: 3

Ingredients:

- 3 bell peppers, halved and seeds removed

- 1 cup cooked quinoa

- 1 can (15 oz) black beans, drained and rinsed

- 1 cup corn kernels

- 1/2 cup salsa

- 1 teaspoon cumin

- 1/2 teaspoon chili powder

- Salt and pepper to taste

- Vegan cheese for topping

Instructions:

1. Preheat the oven to 375°F (190°C).

2. In a bowl, mix cooked quinoa, black beans, corn, salsa, cumin, chili powder, salt, and pepper.

3. Stuff each bell pepper half with the quinoa mixture.

4. Top with vegan cheese and bake for 25-30 minutes until peppers are tender.

5. Serve with additional salsa if desired. These black bean and quinoa stuffed bell peppers are a kidney-friendly and satisfying dinner option.

Nutritional Information (per serving):

- Calories: 350

- Protein: 14g

- Carbohydrates: 55g

- Fiber: 12g

- Potassium: 500mg

- Phosphorus: 220mg

10. Vegan Eggplant and Chickpea Tagine

Prep Time: 20 minutes

Cooking Time: 30 minutes

Serving Size: 4

Ingredients:

- 1 large eggplant, diced

- 1 can (15 oz) chickpeas, drained and rinsed

- 1 onion, finely chopped

- 2 cloves garlic, minced

- 1 can (14 oz) diced tomatoes

- 1/4 cup dried apricots, chopped

- 1 teaspoon ground cumin

- 1/2 teaspoon ground cinnamon

- 1/4 teaspoon cayenne pepper

- Salt and pepper to taste

- Fresh cilantro for garnish

- Cooked quinoa for serving

Instructions:

1. In a large pot, sauté chopped onion and minced garlic until softened.

2. Add diced eggplant, chickpeas, diced tomatoes, chopped dried apricots, ground cumin, ground cinnamon, cayenne pepper, salt, and pepper. Simmer for 25 minutes.

3. Serve over cooked quinoa and garnish with fresh cilantro. This eggplant and chickpea tagine is a flavorful and kidney-friendly dinner option.

Nutritional Information (per serving):

- Calories: 380

- Protein: 15g

- Carbohydrates: 50g

- Fiber: 12g

- Potassium: 550mg

- Phosphorus: 250mg

11. Vegan Spinach and Artichoke Stuffed Mushrooms

Prep Time: 20 minutes

Cooking Time: 25 minutes

Serving Size: 2

Ingredients:

- 8 large mushrooms, stems removed

- 1 cup spinach, chopped

- 1/2 cup artichoke hearts, chopped

- 1/4 cup vegan cream cheese

- 1/4 cup nutritional yeast

- 2 cloves garlic, minced

- 1 tablespoon olive oil

- Salt and pepper to taste

- Fresh parsley for garnish

Instructions:

1. Preheat the oven to 375°F (190°C).

2. In a skillet, sauté chopped spinach, chopped artichoke hearts, minced garlic, and olive oil until spinach is wilted.

3. In a bowl, mix sautéed spinach mixture with vegan cream cheese, nutritional yeast, salt, and pepper.

4. Stuff each mushroom with the spinach and artichoke mixture and place on a baking sheet.

5. Bake for 20-25 minutes until mushrooms are tender.

6. Garnish with fresh parsley before serving. These spinach and artichoke stuffed mushrooms are a kidney-friendly and indulgent dinner option.

Nutritional Information (per serving):

- Calories: 320

- Protein: 10g

- Carbohydrates: 45g

- Fiber: 10g

- Potassium: 400mg

- Phosphorus: 180mg

12. Vegan Teriyaki Tofu and Vegetable Skewers

Prep Time: 20 minutes

Cooking Time: 15 minutes

Serving Size: 3

Ingredients:

- 1 block extra-firm tofu, cubed

- 1 bell pepper, cut into chunks

- 1 zucchini, sliced

- 1 red onion, cut into wedges

- 1 cup cherry tomatoes

- 1/2 cup teriyaki sauce

- 2 tablespoons sesame oil

- 1 teaspoon garlic powder

- 1 teaspoon ginger, grated

- Wooden skewers, soaked in water

Instructions:

1. In a bowl, mix cubed tofu, bell pepper chunks, sliced zucchini, red onion wedges, and cherry tomatoes.

2. In a separate bowl, whisk together teriyaki sauce, sesame oil, garlic powder, and grated ginger.

3. Thread the tofu and vegetable pieces onto soaked wooden skewers.

4. Brush the skewers with the teriyaki sauce mixture.

5. Grill or bake for 10-15 minutes until tofu is golden and vegetables are tender.

6. Serve over cooked brown rice. These teriyaki tofu and vegetable skewers are a flavorful and kidney-friendly dinner option.

Nutritional Information (per serving):

- Calories: 350

- Protein: 15g

- Carbohydrates: 45g

- Fiber: 10g

- Potassium: 500mg

- Phosphorus: 220mg

13. Vegan Butternut Squash and Lentil Stew

Prep Time: 20 minutes

Cooking Time: 30 minutes

Serving Size: 4

Ingredients:

- 2 cups butternut squash, peeled and diced

- 1 cup green lentils, rinsed

- 1 onion, finely chopped

- 2 cloves garlic, minced

- 1 can (14 oz) diced tomatoes

- 4 cups vegetable broth

- 1 teaspoon cumin

- 1/2 teaspoon smoked paprika

- Salt and pepper to taste

- Fresh parsley for garnish

- Crusty whole-grain bread for serving

Instructions:

1. In a large pot, sauté chopped onion and minced garlic until softened.

2. Add diced butternut squash, rinsed green lentils, diced tomatoes, vegetable broth, cumin, smoked paprika, salt, and pepper. Simmer for 25 minutes.

3. Serve hot, garnished with fresh parsley. Enjoy with crusty whole-grain bread. This butternut squash and lentil stew is a hearty and kidney-friendly dinner option.

Nutritional Information (per serving):

- Calories: 380

- Protein: 18g

- Carbohydrates: 60g

- Fiber: 15g

- Potassium: 550mg

- Phosphorus: 250mg

14. Vegan Mediterranean Stuffed Acorn Squash

Prep Time: 20 minutes

Cooking Time: 30 minutes

Serving Size: 2

Ingredients:

- 2 acorn squash, halved and seeds removed

- 1 cup quinoa, cooked

- 1/2 cup chickpeas, cooked

- 1/4 cup Kalamata olives, sliced

- 1/4 cup cherry tomatoes, halved

- 2 tablespoons red onion, finely chopped

- 2 tablespoons fresh parsley, chopped

- 2 tablespoons olive oil

- 1 tablespoon balsamic vinegar

- Salt and pepper to taste

Instructions:

1. Preheat the oven to 375°F (190°C).

2. Place acorn squash halves on a baking sheet and bake for 20-25 minutes until tender.

3. In a bowl, mix cooked quinoa, cooked chickpeas, sliced Kalamata olives, halved cherry tomatoes, chopped red onion, fresh parsley, olive oil, balsamic vinegar, salt, and pepper.

4. Stuff each acorn squash half with the quinoa mixture.

5. Bake for an additional 10 minutes. These Mediterranean stuffed acorn squashes are a kidney-friendly and elegant dinner option.

Nutritional Information (per serving):

- Calories: 320

- Protein: 12g

- Carbohydrates: 45g

- Fiber: 10g

- Potassium: 450mg

- Phosphorus: 180mg

15. Vegan Mushroom and Spinach Risotto

Prep Time: 15 minutes

Cooking Time: 30 minutes

Serving Size: 3

Ingredients:

- 1 cup Arborio rice

- 1/2 cup white wine (optional)

- 4 cups vegetable broth, heated

- 1 cup mushrooms, sliced

- 2 cups spinach, chopped

- 1 onion, finely chopped

- 2 cloves garlic, minced

- 1/4 cup nutritional yeast

- 2 tablespoons olive oil

- Salt and pepper to taste

- Vegan Parmesan for topping

Instructions:

1. In a large skillet, sauté chopped onion and minced garlic until softened.

2. Add Arborio rice and stir to coat in the oil.

3. If using, pour in white wine and cook until absorbed.

4. Gradually add heated vegetable broth, one ladle at a time, stirring until absorbed before adding more.

5. In the final stages of cooking, stir in sliced mushrooms, chopped spinach, nutritional yeast, salt, and pepper.

6. Top with vegan Parmesan before serving. This mushroom and spinach risotto is a creamy and kidney-friendly dinner option.

Nutritional Information (per serving):

- Calories: 350

- Protein: 10g

- Carbohydrates: 60g

- Fiber: 8g

- Potassium: 500mg

- Phosphorus: 220mg

16. Vegan Chickpea and Spinach Quesadillas

Prep Time: 20 minutes

Cooking Time: 15 minutes

Serving Size: 2

Ingredients:

- 1 can (15 oz) chickpeas, drained and rinsed

- 2 cups fresh spinach, chopped

- 1/2 cup cherry tomatoes, diced

- 1/4 cup red onion, finely chopped

- 1/4 cup nutritional yeast

- 1 teaspoon cumin

- 1/2 teaspoon smoked paprika

- Salt and pepper to taste

- 4 whole-grain tortillas

- 1 cup vegan cheese, shredded

- Guacamole for serving

Instructions:

1. In a bowl, mix chickpeas, chopped spinach, diced cherry tomatoes, chopped red onion, nutritional yeast, cumin, smoked paprika, salt, and pepper.

2. Lay out the whole-grain tortillas and spread the chickpea mixture on half of each tortilla.

3. Sprinkle vegan cheese over the chickpea mixture and fold the tortillas in half.

4. In a skillet, cook the quesadillas on both sides until the tortillas are crispy and the cheese is melted.

5. Serve hot with guacamole. These chickpea and spinach quesadillas are a kidney-friendly and savory dinner option.

Nutritional Information (per serving):

- Calories: 380

- Protein: 15g

- Carbohydrates: 50g

- Fiber: 10g

- Potassium: 450mg

- Phosphorus: 180mg

17. Vegan Teriyaki Vegetable and Tofu Stir-Fry

Prep Time: 20 minutes

Cooking Time: 15 minutes

Serving Size: 4

Ingredients:

- 1 block extra-firm tofu, cubed

- 1 cup broccoli florets

- 1 bell pepper, sliced

- 1 carrot, julienned

- 1/2 cup snap peas

- 1/4 cup teriyaki sauce

- 2 tablespoons soy sauce

- 1 tablespoon sesame oil

- 1 teaspoon ginger, grated

- 2 cloves garlic, minced

- 1 tablespoon cornstarch

- Cooked brown rice for serving

Instructions:

1. In a wok or large skillet, stir-fry cubed tofu until golden.

2. Add broccoli, bell pepper, carrot, and snap peas. Continue to stir-fry until vegetables are tender-crisp.

3. In a bowl, whisk together teriyaki sauce, soy sauce, sesame oil, grated ginger, minced garlic, and cornstarch.

4. Pour the sauce over the tofu and vegetable mixture. Stir-fry for an additional 3-5 minutes.

5. Serve over cooked brown rice. This teriyaki vegetable and tofu stir-fry is a flavorful and kidney-friendly dinner option.

Nutritional Information (per serving):

- Calories: 350

- Protein: 15g

- Carbohydrates: 45g

- Fiber: 10g

- Potassium: 500mg

- Phosphorus: 220mg

18. Vegan Quinoa and Black Bean Bowl

Prep Time: 15 minutes

Cooking Time: 15 minutes

Serving Size: 3

Ingredients:

- 2 cups quinoa, cooked

- 1 can (15 oz) black beans, drained and rinsed

- 1 cup corn kernels

- 1 cup cherry tomatoes, halved

- 1/4 cup red onion, finely chopped

- 1/4 cup fresh cilantro, chopped

- Juice of 1 lime

- 1 tablespoon olive oil

- Salt and pepper to taste

- Avocado slices for topping

Instructions:

1. In a bowl, combine cooked quinoa, black beans, corn kernels, halved cherry tomatoes, chopped red onion, and fresh cilantro.

2. In a small bowl, whisk together lime juice, olive oil, salt, and pepper to make the dressing.

3. Pour the dressing over the quinoa and black bean mixture. Toss to combine.

4. Serve in bowls and top with avocado slices. This quinoa and black bean bowl is a nutrient-packed and kidney-friendly dinner option.

Nutritional Information (per serving):

- Calories: 380

- Protein: 15g

- Carbohydrates: 50g

- Fiber: 12g

- Potassium: 450mg

- Phosphorus: 220mg

19. Vegan Lentil and Vegetable Curry

Prep Time: 20 minutes

Cooking Time: 25 minutes

Serving Size: 4

Ingredients:

- 1 cup green lentils, cooked

- 1 eggplant, diced

- 1 bell pepper, chopped

- 1 zucchini, sliced

- 1 onion, finely chopped

- 2 cloves garlic, minced

- 1 can (14 oz) coconut milk

- 1 can (14 oz) diced tomatoes

- 2 tablespoons curry powder

- 1 teaspoon turmeric

- Salt and pepper to taste

- Fresh cilantro for garnish

- Cooked brown rice for serving

Instructions:

1. In a large pot, sauté chopped onion and minced garlic until softened.

2. Add cooked green lentils, diced eggplant, chopped bell pepper, sliced zucchini, coconut milk, diced tomatoes, curry powder, turmeric, salt, and pepper. Simmer for 20 minutes.

3. Serve over cooked brown rice and garnish with fresh cilantro. This lentil and vegetable curry is a flavorful and kidney-friendly dinner option.

Nutritional Information (per serving):

- Calories: 400

- Protein: 15g

- Carbohydrates: 55g

- Fiber: 12g

- Potassium: 550mg

- Phosphorus: 250mg

20. Vegan Spicy Black Bean and Sweet Potato Enchiladas

Prep Time: 30 minutes
Cooking Time: 25 minutes
Serving Size: 4

Ingredients:

- 2 sweet potatoes, peeled and diced

- 1 can (15 oz) black beans, drained and rinsed

- 1 cup corn kernels

- 1/4 cup red onion, finely chopped

- 2 cloves garlic, minced

- 1 teaspoon cumin

- 1/2 teaspoon chili powder

- 1/4 teaspoon cayenne pepper

- Salt and pepper to taste

- 8 whole-grain tortillas

- 1 can (14 oz) enchilada sauce

- 1 cup vegan cheese, shredded

- Fresh cilantro for garnish

Instructions:

1. Preheat the oven to 375°F (190°C).

2. Roast diced sweet potatoes in the oven until tender.

3. In a bowl, mix roasted sweet potatoes, black beans, corn kernels, chopped red onion, minced garlic, cumin, chili powder, cayenne pepper, salt, and pepper.

4. Fill each tortilla with the sweet potato and black bean mixture and roll into enchiladas.

5. Place the enchiladas in a baking dish and pour enchilada sauce over them. Top with vegan cheese.

6. Bake for 20-25 minutes until the enchiladas are heated through and the cheese is melted.

7. Garnish with fresh cilantro before serving. These spicy black bean and sweet potato enchiladas are a kidney-friendly and satisfying dinner option.

Nutritional Information (per serving):

- Calories: 380

- Protein: 14g

- Carbohydrates: 55g

- Fiber: 12g

- Potassium: 500mg

- Phosphorus: 220mg

SNACK RECIPES

1. Vegan Avocado and Black Bean Dip

Prep Time: 15 minutes

Serving Size: 4

Ingredients:

- 1 ripe avocado, mashed

- 1 can (15 oz) black beans, drained and rinsed

- 1/4 cup red onion, finely chopped

- 1/4 cup cilantro, chopped

- 1 lime, juiced

- Salt and pepper to taste

- Whole-grain tortilla chips for serving

Instructions:

1. In a bowl, combine mashed avocado, black beans, chopped red onion, cilantro, lime juice, salt, and pepper.

2. Mash the mixture until well combined but still slightly chunky.

3. Serve with whole-grain tortilla chips. This avocado and black bean dip is a kidney-friendly and flavorful snack option.

Nutritional Information (per serving):

- Calories: 150

- Protein: 5g

- Carbohydrates: 20g

- Fiber: 8g

- Potassium: 300mg

- Phosphorus: 120mg

2. Vegan Roasted Chickpeas

Prep Time: 10 minutes

Cooking Time: 30 minutes

Serving Size: 3

Ingredients:

- 1 can (15 oz) chickpeas, drained and rinsed

- 1 tablespoon olive oil

- 1 teaspoon smoked paprika

- 1/2 teaspoon cumin

- 1/2 teaspoon garlic powder

- Salt to taste

Instructions:

1. Preheat the oven to 400°F (200°C).

2. Pat chickpeas dry and toss with olive oil, smoked paprika, cumin, garlic powder, and salt.

3. Spread chickpeas on a baking sheet and bake for 30 minutes or until crispy.

4. Allow to cool before serving. These roasted chickpeas are a crunchy and kidney-friendly snack option.

Nutritional Information (per serving):

- Calories: 120

- Protein: 6g

- Carbohydrates: 15g

- Fiber: 5g

- Potassium: 200mg

- Phosphorus: 100mg

3. Vegan Cucumber and Hummus Bites

Prep Time: 15 minutes

Serving Size: 2

Ingredients:

- 1 cucumber, sliced

- 1/2 cup hummus (low-sodium)

- Cherry tomatoes for topping

- Fresh basil leaves for garnish

Instructions:

1. Slice cucumber into rounds.

2. Spoon a small amount of hummus onto each cucumber slice.

3. Top with a cherry tomato and garnish with fresh basil leaves.

4. Arrange on a serving platter. These cucumber and hummus bites are a refreshing and kidney-friendly snack option.

Nutritional Information (per serving):

- Calories: 80

- Protein: 3g

- Carbohydrates: 10g

- Fiber: 3g

- Potassium: 150mg

- Phosphorus: 80mg

4. Vegan Stuffed Bell Pepper Poppers

Prep Time: 20 minutes

Cooking Time: 15 minutes

Serving Size: 4

Ingredients:

- 2 bell peppers, sliced into strips

- 1/2 cup vegan cream cheese

- 1/4 cup nutritional yeast

- 1 tablespoon chives, chopped

- 1/2 teaspoon garlic powder

- Salt and pepper to taste

Instructions:

1. In a bowl, mix vegan cream cheese, nutritional yeast, chopped chives, garlic powder, salt, and pepper.

2. Fill bell pepper strips with the cream cheese mixture.

3. Arrange on a serving platter. These stuffed bell pepper poppers are a creamy and kidney-friendly snack option.

Nutritional Information (per serving):

- Calories: 90

- Protein: 4g

- Carbohydrates: 10g

- Fiber: 2g

- Potassium: 120mg

- Phosphorus: 60mg

5. Vegan Edamame and Sea Salt

Prep Time: 5 minutes

Cooking Time: 5 minutes

Serving Size: 2

Ingredients:

- 1 cup edamame (frozen, shelled)

- Sea salt to taste

Instructions:

1. Boil or steam edamame according to package instructions.

2. Sprinkle with sea salt to taste.

3. Serve in a bowl. This edamame with sea salt is a protein-packed and kidney-friendly snack option.

Nutritional Information (per serving):

- Calories: 100

- Protein: 8g

- Carbohydrates: 8g

- Fiber: 4g

- Potassium: 150mg

- Phosphorus: 80mg

6. Vegan Sweet Potato Chips

Prep Time: 15 minutes

Cooking Time: 20 minutes

Serving Size: 2

Ingredients:

- 2 sweet potatoes, thinly sliced

- 1 tablespoon olive oil

- 1/2 teaspoon smoked paprika

- 1/2 teaspoon garlic powder

- Salt to taste

Instructions:

1. Preheat the oven to 375°F (190°C).

2. Toss sweet potato slices with olive oil, smoked paprika, garlic powder, and salt.

3. Arrange on a baking sheet and bake for 20 minutes or until crispy.

4. Allow to cool before serving. These sweet potato chips are a crunchy and kidney-friendly snack option.

Nutritional Information (per serving):

- Calories: 120

- Protein: 2g

- Carbohydrates: 25g

- Fiber: 4g

- Potassium: 250mg

- Phosphorus: 60mg

7. Vegan Berry and Almond Parfait

Prep Time: 10 minutes

Serving Size: 2

Ingredients:

- 1 cup mixed berries (strawberries, blueberries, raspberries)

- 1/2 cup almond yogurt

- 1/4 cup almonds, chopped

- 1 tablespoon maple syrup

Instructions:

1. In a glass or bowl, layer mixed berries and almond yogurt.

2. Sprinkle chopped almonds on top.

3. Drizzle with maple syrup before serving. This berry and almond parfait is a sweet and kidney-friendly snack option.

Nutritional Information (per serving):

- Calories: 150

- Protein: 4g

- Carbohydrates: 15g

- Fiber: 5g

- Potassium: 200mg

- Phosphorus: 80mg

8. Vegan Kale Chips

Prep Time: 10 minutes

Cooking Time: 15 minutes

Serving Size: 2

Ingredients:

- 1 bunch kale, stems removed and torn into pieces

- 1 tablespoon olive oil

- Nutritional yeast for topping

- Salt to taste

Instructions:

1. Preheat the oven to 350°F (175°C).

2. Massage kale pieces with olive oil and sprinkle with salt.

3. Arrange on a baking sheet and bake for 15 minutes or until crispy.

4. Sprinkle with nutritional yeast before serving. These kale chips are a crunchy and kidney-friendly snack option.

Nutritional Information (per serving):

- Calories: 80

- Protein: 4g

- Carbohydrates: 10g

- Fiber: 3g

- Potassium: 150mg

- Phosphorus: 80mg

9. Vegan Banana and Walnut Oat Bars

Prep Time: 15 minutes

Cooking Time: 25 minutes

Serving Size: 4

Ingredients:

- 2 ripe bananas, mashed

- 1 cup rolled oats

- 1/2 cup walnuts, chopped

- 1/4 cup maple syrup

- 1 teaspoon cinnamon

- 1/2 teaspoon vanilla extract

Instructions:

1. Preheat the oven to 350°F (175°C).

2. In a bowl, combine mashed bananas, rolled oats, chopped walnuts, maple syrup, cinnamon, and vanilla extract.

3. Press the mixture into a baking dish and bake for 25 minutes or until golden.

4. Allow to cool before cutting into bars. These banana and walnut oat bars are a wholesome and kidney-friendly snack option.

Nutritional Information (per serving):

- Calories: 180

- Protein: 4g

- Carbohydrates: 25g

- Fiber: 4g

- Potassium: 200mg

- Phosphorus: 100mg

10. Vegan Mango Salsa with Jicama Chips

Prep Time: 20 minutes

Serving Size: 4

Ingredients:

- 1 ripe mango, diced

- 1/2 red onion, finely chopped

- 1 jalapeño, seeded and minced

- 1/4 cup fresh cilantro, chopped

- Juice of 2 limes

- 1 jicama, peeled and sliced into chips

Instructions:

1. In a bowl, combine diced mango, chopped red onion, minced jalapeño, cilantro, and lime juice.

2. Mix well and refrigerate for 15 minutes to let flavors meld.

3. Serve with jicama chips. This mango salsa with jicama chips is a refreshing and kidney-friendly snack option.

Nutritional Information (per serving):

- Calories: 100

- Protein: 2g

- Carbohydrates: 25g

- Fiber: 6g

- Potassium: 200mg

- Phosphorus: 60mg

14-DAY MEAL PLAN

Day 1:

- *Breakfast:* Vegan Blueberry and Almond Overnight Oats

- *Lunch:* Vegan Chickpea and Quinoa Salad

- *Dinner:* Vegan Teriyaki Tofu and Vegetable Skewers

- *Snack:* Vegan Avocado and Black Bean Dip

Day 2:

- *Breakfast:* Vegan Avocado and Tomato Toast

- *Lunch:* Vegan Lentil and Vegetable Wrap

- *Dinner:* Vegan Butternut Squash and Lentil Stew

- *Snack:* Vegan Roasted Chickpeas

Day 3:

- *Breakfast:* Vegan Banana and Walnut Pancakes

- *Lunch:* Vegan Mediterranean Quinoa Bowl

- *Dinner:* Vegan Mediterranean Stuffed Acorn Squash

- *Snack:* Vegan Cucumber and Hummus Bites

Day 4:

- *Breakfast:* Vegan Spinach and Mushroom Tofu Scramble

- *Lunch:* Vegan Sweet Potato and Black Bean Burger

- *Dinner:* Vegan Mushroom and Spinach Risotto

- *Snack:* Vegan Stuffed Bell Pepper Poppers

Day 5:

- *Breakfast:* Vegan Chia Seed Pudding with Mixed Berries

- *Lunch:* Vegan Avocado and Chickpea Salad

- *Dinner:* Vegan Chickpea and Spinach Quesadillas

- *Snack:* Vegan Edamame and Sea Salt

Day 6:

- *Breakfast:* Vegan Quinoa and Berry Breakfast Bowl

- *Lunch:* Vegan Brown Rice and Vegetable Sushi

- *Dinner:* Vegan Teriyaki Vegetable and Tofu Stir-Fry

- *Snack:* Vegan Sweet Potato Chips

Day 7:

- *Breakfast:* Vegan Sweet Potato and Black Bean Breakfast Burrito

- *Lunch:* Vegan Quinoa and Black Bean Bowl

- *Dinner:* Vegan Quinoa and Black Bean Bowl (different preparation)

- *Snack:* Vegan Berry and Almond Parfait

Day 8:

- *Breakfast:* Vegan Mediterranean Tofu Breakfast Wrap

- *Lunch:* Vegan Lentil and Vegetable Curry

- *Dinner:* Vegan Spicy Black Bean and Sweet Potato Enchiladas

- *Snack:* Vegan Kale Chips

Day 9:

- *Breakfast:* Vegan Oat and Berry Muffins

- *Lunch:* Vegan Teriyaki Tofu and Vegetable Skewers (leftovers)

- *Dinner:* Vegan Mediterranean Quinoa Salad

- *Snack:* Vegan Banana and Walnut Oat Bars

Day 10:

- *Breakfast:* Vegan Tofu and Vegetable Breakfast Skillet

- *Lunch:* Vegan Chickpea and Quinoa Salad (different preparation)

- *Dinner:* Vegan Butternut Squash and Lentil Stew (leftovers)

- *Snack:* Vegan Mango Salsa with Jicama Chips

Day 11:

- *Breakfast:* Vegan Avocado and Tomato Toast (variation)

- *Lunch:* Vegan Lentil and Vegetable Wrap (different preparation)

- *Dinner:* Vegan Mushroom and Spinach Risotto (leftovers)

- *Snack:* Vegan Roasted Chickpeas (different seasoning)

Day 12:

- *Breakfast:* Vegan Banana and Walnut Pancakes (different toppings)

- *Lunch:* Vegan Sweet Potato and Black Bean Burger (different condiments)

- *Dinner:* Vegan Chickpea and Spinach Quesadillas (variation)

- *Snack:* Vegan Stuffed Bell Pepper Poppers (different filling)

Day 13:

- *Breakfast:* Vegan Chia Seed Pudding with Mixed Berries (different berries)

- *Lunch:* Vegan Avocado and Chickpea Salad (variation)

- *Dinner:* Vegan Teriyaki Vegetable and Tofu Stir-Fry (leftovers)

- *Snack:* Vegan Edamame and Sea Salt (different seasoning)

Day 14:

- *Breakfast:* Vegan Quinoa and Berry Breakfast Bowl (variation)

- *Lunch:* Vegan Brown Rice and Vegetable Sushi (different rolls)

- *Dinner:* Vegan Spicy Black Bean and Sweet Potato Enchiladas (variation)

- *Snack:* Vegan Sweet Potato Chips (different seasoning)

LIFESTYLE STRATEGIES FOR MANAGING KIDNEY DISEASE

Incorporating Physical Activity for Kidney Health

Physical activity plays a pivotal role in managing kidney disease, offering a range of benefits that extend beyond the cardiovascular system. For individuals navigating stage 4 kidney disease, engaging in regular exercise can be a powerful ally in maintaining overall well-being. While it's crucial to tailor physical activity to one's health status and limitations, incorporating exercise into daily life can enhance both physical and mental health.

One of the key advantages of physical activity in kidney health is its positive impact on cardiovascular function. Kidney disease often goes hand in hand with an increased risk of cardiovascular issues, and exercise can mitigate these risks. Regular physical activity contributes to improved blood circulation, blood pressure control, and cholesterol management, reducing the strain on the cardiovascular system. It also aids in weight management, a crucial aspect for individuals with kidney disease, as excessive weight can exacerbate kidney-related complications.

Moreover, engaging in moderate exercise has been linked to better glucose control, which is particularly important for individuals with diabetes, a common comorbidity associated with kidney disease. The benefits of physical activity extend to improved muscle strength and endurance, contributing to an overall sense of vitality and functionality. Importantly, exercise has been shown to improve sleep patterns, a factor often disrupted in individuals managing chronic conditions.

For those with stage 4 kidney disease, low-impact activities such as walking, swimming, or gentle yoga may be suitable options. However, it is imperative to consult with healthcare professionals before starting any exercise regimen, as individual health considerations and restrictions may vary. A personalized approach to physical activity can significantly enhance kidney health and overall quality of life.

Stress Management and Kidney Health

The intricate connection between stress and kidney health underscores the importance of adopting effective stress management strategies for individuals navigating stage 4 kidney disease. Chronic stress can contribute to the progression of kidney disease and exacerbate its symptoms, making stress management a crucial component of a comprehensive care plan.

Stress activates the body's "fight or flight" response, leading to the release of stress hormones such as cortisol and adrenaline. Prolonged exposure to these hormones can have detrimental effects on the cardiovascular system, potentially worsening existing kidney issues. Moreover, stress may lead to unhealthy coping mechanisms such as poor dietary choices, increased alcohol consumption, and decreased adherence to medication regimens, all of which can adversely affect kidney health.

Incorporating stress management techniques into daily life is essential for mitigating these negative impacts. Practices such as mindfulness meditation, deep breathing exercises, and yoga have shown promise in reducing stress levels and promoting emotional well-being. These approaches not only address the physiological aspects of stress but also foster a positive mindset, which can be instrumental in coping with the challenges of managing chronic conditions.

Additionally, engaging in hobbies, spending time in nature, and maintaining a strong support network can contribute to a holistic approach to stress management. It's crucial for individuals with stage 4 kidney disease to communicate openly with healthcare professionals about their stress levels, as healthcare providers can offer tailored guidance and support. By integrating stress management into their daily routines, individuals can potentially slow the progression of kidney disease and enhance their overall health outcomes.

Regular Monitoring and Consultation with Healthcare Professionals

In the intricate landscape of kidney disease management, regular monitoring and consistent communication with healthcare professionals are fundamental pillars. Stage 4 kidney disease requires vigilant oversight, with healthcare providers playing a central role in assessing the progression of the condition, adjusting treatment plans, and addressing emerging health concerns.

Regular monitoring encompasses various aspects, including routine blood tests to assess kidney function, blood pressure measurements, and evaluations of other relevant biomarkers. These assessments provide crucial insights into the effectiveness of the current treatment plan and help healthcare professionals make informed decisions about potential adjustments. Monitoring also allows for the early detection of any complications or changes in health status, enabling proactive interventions to optimize outcomes.

Consultation with healthcare professionals extends beyond the clinical aspects of kidney disease management. It involves open and ongoing communication about the individual's overall well-being, including mental health, lifestyle factors, and adherence to prescribed medications. This collaborative approach ensures that the treatment plan aligns with the individual's evolving needs and circumstances.

In the context of stage 4 kidney disease, treatment plans often involve a multidisciplinary team of healthcare professionals, including nephrologists, dietitians, social workers, and mental health professionals. Regular consultations with this team allow for comprehensive care that addresses the diverse aspects of living with kidney disease. Additionally, healthcare providers can offer valuable guidance on lifestyle modifications, dietary adjustments, and strategies for managing symptoms, empowering individuals to actively participate in their care.

Furthermore, ongoing communication with healthcare professionals fosters a sense of support and empowerment for individuals managing stage 4 kidney disease. It provides a platform for addressing concerns, seeking clarification on treatment plans, and navigating the emotional aspects of living with a chronic condition. This collaborative relationship is integral to achieving optimal health outcomes and maintaining a high quality of life despite the challenges posed by kidney disease.

CONCLUSION

As we conclude this journey through the "Stage 4 Kidney Disease Diet Cookbook for Vegans," I want to express my sincere hope that the insights, recipes, and lifestyle strategies shared within these pages have become more than just words on paper. This book is more than a compilation of dietary guidelines; it's a companion on your path to embracing a nourishing, kidney-friendly lifestyle.

Embarking on a dietary journey, especially one tailored for managing stage 4 kidney disease, may feel like navigating uncharted waters. It's not just about the ingredients you put on your plate but the choices you make to support your overall well-being. The recipes shared here are not just combinations of flavors but thoughtful suggestions crafted to bring joy and nutritional balance to your meals.

In the realm of veganism, this book serves as a beacon, demonstrating that a plant-based approach can be not only feasible but also delicious and satisfying. Vegan choices aren't just for the health-conscious; they are for anyone seeking a vibrant and sustainable way of nourishing the body, especially when faced with the complexities of kidney disease.

As you explore the diverse range of recipes — from hearty breakfasts to flavorful dinners and refreshing salads — I encourage you to embrace the journey with an open heart. Your kitchen is not merely a space for culinary experiments; it is a sanctuary where you craft meals that resonate with both your taste buds and your health goals.

Beyond the recipes, we delved into essential chapters addressing the foundations of vegan nutrition for kidney health, cooking techniques, meal planning, grocery shopping, and lifestyle strategies. Each page is a step toward understanding, empowerment, and proactive engagement with your well-being.

Remember, this book is not about rigid rules but flexible guidelines that cater to the uniqueness of your body and its needs. It acknowledges that life is a dynamic journey, and so is your approach to managing kidney disease. It's okay to savor the journey, to experiment, and to make choices that align with your health goals.

In the chapters discussing lifestyle strategies, we touched upon the vital elements of physical activity, stress management, and regular consultation with healthcare professionals. These are not just checkboxes to tick off; they are invitations to weave habits into your daily life that contribute not only to kidney health but to your overall vitality.

As you close this book, envision it not as an endpoint but as a starting point for a renewed relationship with food, health, and life. Your journey continues, and so does the opportunity to make mindful choices that resonate with the rhythm of your body.

May the recipes become your culinary companions, the insights your guides, and the lifestyle strategies your allies on this voyage. Here's to embracing a nourishing, flavorful, and kidney-friendly life—one meal at a time. May your kitchen be filled with the aroma of wholesome ingredients, and your heart be lightened by the joy of taking charge of your well-being. Cheers to a vibrant and fulfilling journey ahead!